MUDPACKS AI

Experiencing Ayurvedic, Biomedical and Religious Healing

MURPHY HALLIBURTON

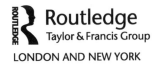

Routledge
Taylor & Francis Group

LONDON AND NEW YORK

First published 2009 by Left Coast Press, Inc.

Published 2016 by Routledge
2 Park Square, Milton Park, Abingdon, Oxon OX14 4RN
711 Third Avenue, New York, NY 10017, USA

Routledge is an imprint of the Taylor & Francis Group, an informa business

Copyright © 2009 Taylor & Francis

Library of Congress Cataloging-in-Publication Data

Halliburton, Murphy, 1964-
  Mudpacks and prozac : experiencing Ayurvedic, biomedical, and religious healing / Murphy Halliburton.
    p. cm.
Includes bibliographical references and index.
ISBN 978-1-59874-398-2 (hardcover : alk. paper)—ISBN 978-1-59874-399-9 (pbk. : alk. paper)
1. Traditional medicine—India—Kerala. 2. Cultural psychiatry—India—Kerala.
3. Medicine, Ayurvedic—India—Kerala. 4. Healing—Social aspects—India—Kerala.
5. Human mechanics—India—Kerala. 6. Kerala (India)—Social life and customs.
I. Title.

 GR305.5.K4H35 2009
 954'.83—dc22
 2009019105

Cover design by Hannah Jennings

Hardback ISBN 978-1-59874-398-2
Paperback ISBN 978-1-59874-399-9

MUDPACKS AND PROZAC

For **Amy, Luca** and **Sophie**

and

The people suffering mental distress

who shared their stories with me.

May they find some relief.

CONTENTS

ACKNOWLEDGMENTS

Many people helped with the design, development and completion of this project, and unfortunately I will only be able to name a few here. I first acknowledge my debt to my mentors at the Department of Anthropology of the City University of New York (CUNY) Graduate Center, Vincent Crapanzano, Shirley Lindenbaum, Joan Mencher and Setha Low. Equally crucial to this endeavor was the generous assistance of many in the mental health field in Kerala, India. This project would truly not have been possible without the tireless assistance and devoted friendship of Dr. K. Gireesh, clinical psychologist of the Trivandrum Mental Health Centre. Also fundamental to my fieldwork efforts and the development of my knowledge of health and healing are Dr. V. George Mathew (Department of Psychology, University of Kerala), Dr. K. Sundaran (Government Ayurveda Mental Hospital, Kottakkal), Dr. John Baby (Department of Psychology, University of Calicut) and Dr. K. A. Kumar (Trivandrum Medical College Hospital). I am also greatly indebted to my research assistants, Kavitha N. S., T.R. "Biju" Bijumohan and Benny Verghese for their insights and service and for making the research process so much more enjoyable. Meanwhile, for making the early phases of this project a more pleasant process, I am grateful for the support of Hugo Benavides, Aseel Sawalha, Jonathan Shannon, Molly Doane, Kee Yong and Alcira Forero-Peña. Earlier versions of this manuscript benefited greatly from the insights of Thomas Csordas, Michael Nunley and Kevin Birth and the thorough and thoughtful work of the anonymous reviewers of this project. Finally, I profoundly appreciate the enthusiastic, hard-working staff of Left Coast Press, especially their insightful and encouraging senior editor Jennifer Collier, for their efforts and support.

Research for this project was made possible by grants from the Wenner Gren Foundation for Anthropological Research and the National Science Foundation. Some material and ideas in Chapter 4 first appeared in my article "Rethinking Anthropological Studies of the Body: Manas and Bodham in Kerala." *American Anthropologist* 104(4): 1123–1134, December 2002. Parts of Chapter 5 and some basic ideas in this work were first developed in "The Importance of a Pleasant Process of Treatment: Lessons on Healing from South India." *Culture, Medicine and Psychiatry* 27: 161–186, June 2003.

1

INTRODUCTION

When I met "Ajit" in an ayurvedic hospital in Kerala, India, he had already tried two of the most popular therapies for mental illness. Seeking relief from emotional distress, sleeplessness and violent outbursts, he underwent the medicated mudpack treatments of ayurvedic psychiatry, which is based on the South Asian system of medical practices known as *ayurveda*. He had also used the psychoactive pharmaceuticals of Western biomedical psychiatry, which is known in India as "allopathy" or, in a phrase evocative of allopathy's colonial origins, "English medicine." Ajit had not visited any of the religious sites that are also reputed as healing centers for people with mental health problems, but the young man had recently participated in a pilgrimage, which he feels helped him achieve some mental peace.

During our first encounter Ajit offered an impassioned discourse on the ideals and practices of ayurvedic and allopathic medicine in the changing context of health in "modern society":[1]

> In the case of allopathic doctors, after asking two or three questions, they will know which medicine to prescribe. But ayurvedic doctors, they want to take the patient to another level. At that level, things are very different. Right now I am taking treatment for mental illness. For this illness, there is a painful method. It is giving "shocks." After going there and coming here [referring to allopathy and ayurveda], I feel this is better. But now everyone "prefers modern medicine." It is because of "modern society" that some are reluctant to come to ayurveda.[2]

There might be some good aspects in allopathy when one looks at its research and other things, but if we want to get good coolness [*kulirmma*], if we want to reach a good goal [*nalla lakshyam*] . . . Right now, speaking about our life, what is it? If I have a fever, I must get better [literally, must get changed—*māranam*]. For what? To go to work the next day. Get a cold, get changed [*māranam*] in order to go to school the next day. This is the level at which we maintain our health. If we have a supreme aim in life, ayurveda will help us attain it.

These brief but insightful comments, like those of many other patients I met, delve directly into phenomenology and the nature of embodiment, issues that captivate me as a medical anthropologist. Most notably, the aesthetic experience of medical treatment is a central concern for the patients I interviewed. Ajit specifically comments here on the visceral experience of different therapies. Giving "shocks," or electroconvulsive therapy, he considers painful, whereas he reports that his "head got cooled" from ayurvedic therapy, evoking a local idiom for a pleasant aesthetic effect. I found that similar experiences were recounted by other people suffering mental afflictions in Kerala, many of whom abandoned allopathic psychiatric treatment to pursue a different form of healing because of what they experienced as uncomfortable or abrasive methods of treatment. Whereas allopathy may involve an occasionally painful healing process, patients report that ayurveda usually provides less abrasive and, at times, aesthetically pleasant therapeutic experiences. Ajit employs the Malayalam term *kulirmma*, which translates roughly as "coolness" and "satisfaction," to describe the aesthetic experience he obtained through ayurvedic treatment.

On one level, it seems perfectly obvious that patients would be concerned with the pain or pleasure they experience. And yet, the ways in which the aesthetic pleasantness of treatments differ between medical systems have been overlooked in studies of mental healing. Scholars tend not to take aesthetic pleasantness seriously either as a source of insight about concepts such as embodiment, healing and curing, or as a source of insight into critical public health issues such as how and why patients seek treatments, make decisions about treatments, and navigate multiple medical systems. The seemingly mundane fact that patients tend to prefer a therapy that feels good—or is "cooling," as they say in South India—over one that is more abrasive or painful is actually a rich point of departure for medical anthropological inquiry.

In investigating aesthetics, I am also concerned with experiences that run much deeper than simple pleasure or pain. In the preceding quote, Ajit also claims that ayurvedic doctors attempt to bring the patient to "another level," a positive transformation he alleges can occur through ayurvedic therapy. This also evokes the experience of people who seek religious therapies at temples, mosques and churches, where they undergo aesthetically rich healing processes that engage the senses through music, smells and a scenic environment. Although many report only moderate improvement after therapy, some recount undergoing a transformative process that brought them to a state similar to what Ajit describes, a level of well-being that is more vibrant than the normal "healthy" state they experienced before their illness. Here *health* does not signify merely an absence of illness—it is not merely "remedial," to borrow Alter's (1999) label for contemporary biomedical and social science assumptions about health. Rather, it is something that can be continually improved upon or "changed," as they say in Kerala when describing what is accomplished in healing.

An awareness of the pleasantness of the process of healing thus leads to a recognition of the contingency of *time* in healing and the limitations of the concept of *curing* for understanding what is accomplished in therapy. There is no word in Malayalam, the primary language of Kerala, that has quite the same meaning as the English term "cure" or that depicts the allopathic orientation to treatment. Curing implies an eradication of a pathogen or a return to a state of normalcy, or a "baseline," that existed prior to an illness. "Cure" is in some contexts more ideal or ambitious than the verb *māruka*, meaning "change" (or, more loosely, "improve," "get better"), which is used in Kerala to describe the improvement one attains through therapy. The concept of "curing," or even "healing," meanwhile, falls short of capturing the sense of moving to a higher level or the auspicious transformation reported by some who were using religious therapies.

Since people in Kerala have several, mainstream therapeutic options, many patients discontinue unpleasant treatments to pursue less abrasive forms of healing. Some people with intractable mental illnesses that have persisted for years have found a "solution" to their problems, not in achieving a cure, but in resolving to live with their problems in the aesthetically and spiritually engaging environment of a religious healing center. In other words, they have decided to live *in* a process of therapy that is "pleasant" in the sense of being positively aesthetically engaging and where the contingency of time is de-emphasized. The concern about the aesthetic quality of the process of therapy in ayurveda and the actions of those who choose to live with their problems in a religious center suggest an orientation to the process and goals of therapy that is less teleological, less oriented to absolute endings than the orientation in allopathic medical practice. Both approaches involve working toward goals, but the ayurvedic and religious orientations attend to the quality of the present—the process—while moving forward, whereas allopathic therapy proceeds with a more emphatic focus on the future and with a concern that results should come quickly. Recall that Ajit described allopathic psychiatric treatment as having a "sudden effect." Although allopathic treatment does not attend as much to the quality of the present—that is, the process of therapy—the speed of allopathic therapy appeals to people who feel they do not have time to engage in gentler but slower ayurvedic treatment.

Ajit calls our attention to another aspect of the aesthetic and phenomenological experience of illness when he describes his problem as a "mental" (*manasika*) illness. "Mental" is one of several idioms, including *bōdham* ("consciousness") and *ōrmma* ("consciousness/memory"), which people in Kerala use to describe their experiences of illness. These idioms, and the modes of experience they represent, form part of a local phenomenological orientation, a set of relations between mind, body, consciousness and other parts of the person through which one mediates one's experience of the world. I describe this as a "local" phenomenological orientation because I am suggesting that these orientations are culturally and historically constructed. "Local" phenomenologies are, of course, informed by larger discourses and philosophies, but as opposed to a universal phenomenology, which philosophers have long attempted to define, people suffering "mental" distress in south India reveal that people experience the world through a variety of phenomenologies. People in various settings make sense of their personhood and their way of being in the world in terms of a range of modes of experience and perception—mind, *manas,* body, *ōrmma,* soi, dasein, among others—that cannot be reduced to mind-body dualism or embodiment.

In anthropology, cultural studies, philosophy, gender studies and other fields, much attention has been paid to the paradigm of embodiment and to intriguing critiques of the limitations of Western mind-body dualism. For a long period, perhaps since the development of modern research universities, academic enquiry focused almost exclusively on thought and mental representation, overlooking how people feel and experience the world viscerally or through the body. To correct this representationalist bias, researchers over the last two decades have examined how our embodied experience shapes our engagement with the world and have questioned what they see as the limitations of mind-body dualism. Ethnographers claimed to have found peoples who transcend the dichotomies of western mind-body dualism and ground experience more firmly in the body, a discovery that actually continues a long-term trend in Western academia to find in the East or the cultural Other the fulfillment of what is lacking in modernity and the West. The search for the embodied Other, in which research on the body appears to be caught, has led us to overlook what may be a great diversity of phenomenological experience that cultures construct differently in various settings. Living neither in the realm of Descartes and Heidegger nor in a grounded, embodied alternative, people in Kerala distinguish between body, mind, *buddhi* ("intellect"), *bōdham* ("consciousness"), *ōrmma* ("consciousness/memory"), and *ātman* ("the true, essential self"), idioms that are found in Indian philosophical and religious texts and that are used by people whom I spoke with in Kerala. These particular idioms constitute a continuum of increasingly intangible modes of experience—from the highly tangible body to the completely intangible *ātman*—in which the more intangible realms are more highly valued.

The nature of the aesthetic quality of healing and the phenomenological orientation reflected in the experience of people suffering illness in Kerala are historically contingent to a certain degree, and they continually encounter and counter various influences. There is evidence that in the past, more invasive and painful procedures existed in ayurveda along with gentler methods of treatment, but ayurvedic practitioners now place greater emphasis on less invasive, nonviolent methods to distinguish their practice from allopathic medicine (Zimmermann 1992). Meanwhile, people in Kerala are reporting increasing time pressure due to contemporary work regimens with the consequence that they say they have less time to undergo these lengthier, nonabrasive therapies. While Ajit says that ayurvedic doctors want to take people to a higher level, he also explains that today when one is ill one must get over it quickly in order to get back to work or school. Ayurvedic therapy can take weeks, but, as Ajit observes, an allopathic doctor prescribes a pill after asking two or three questions. In addition, the proliferation of allopathic psychiatric and psychological discourses in the media and in popular culture corresponds to alterations in "idioms of distress" in Kerala.[3] More people are complaining of problems like "tension" or "depression" and using these English terms to describe their afflictions. These Western, embodied depictions of mental states may be modifying the phenomenological orientations people engage with in South India.

Embodiment and Phenomenology

Interpretations that seek explicitly to collapse mind/body dualities, or that are essentially dialectical or montage-like in form, are now privileged. The body is no longer portrayed simply as a template for social organization, nor as a biological black box cut off from "mind," and nature/culture and mind/body dualities are self-consciously interrogated (Lock 1993: 136).

This observation by Margaret Lock in 1993 describes a turn to the body in the 1980s and 1990s in fields ranging from anthropology to comparative literature. This transition provided a profound corrective to studies that looked at human experience in cognitive or mentalistic terms and through the assumptions of Western mind-body dualism. Until the late twentieth century, researchers and scholars overemphasized the realm of the mind, focusing on concepts, ideas and representations of human experience while paying little attention to visceral experience, the world of the senses, or the fact that our perception is shaped by our condition of being in a body.[4]

The discovery of the body and embodied experience profoundly affects social and cultural analyses of health and illness. Illness is a powerfully embodied experience that was previously approached by medical anthropologists and other social scientists in terms of peoples' concepts and beliefs.[5] While different people, or cultures, may have different "understandings" of the body or "concepts" about healing and the "meaning" of illness, illness and healing are highly embodied experiences. They are not just conceived: they are felt, lived, and experienced, affecting the person bodily, aesthetically and emotionally as well as mentally and existentially. In examining experiences of illness and healing in India, I am both embracing and refining this turn to the body. I consider the importance of the aesthetic-experiential realm for comprehending the process of healing while going beyond the depiction of non-Western subjects as people who are somehow more in touch with their bodies to depict a greater variety of aesthetic and phenomenological orientations than we previously imagined.

While drawing our attention to the body, researchers have created a picture of the world wherein peoples who are labeled "non-Western" or "traditional" are either more grounded in their bodies or they experience the world with a more subtle awareness of mind-body interconnection.[6] Meanwhile we are led to imagine that the Western subject is naively unaware of the embodied nature of his own experience (I say "his" intentionally; the Western woman is frequently seen as akin to the non-Western subject in her awareness of her body). "Mental" patients and spirit-possessed people in Kerala, however, express their suffering explicitly in terms of the mind and other intangible parts of the person, which I suggest actually represents a greater degree of rarification away from the body, or a more fine-tuned parsing of the intangible from the material, than is contained in Western mind-body phenomenology.

Attempting to discern and map out local phenomenologies, orientations to experience, which are not simply about the body but about the condition in which a person lives as a combination of mind, body and other locally construed modes of experience, should provide richer insights into the nature of human experience than our tendency to look for transcendence of Western mind-body dualism in the world outside the modern, middle-class West.

Having leaned on the term "phenomenology" at several points already, I should explain that this term has multiple and ambiguous meanings, and I should clarify how I am using it. There is no succinct or consensus definition of "phenomenology." The term is associated with the philosophy of Husserl, Hegel, Heidegger and Merleau-Ponty, among other Western thinkers. Also, diverse movements within Buddhist, Japanese, Indian and other cultures and philosophies have been considered phenomenological. Phenomenology is concerned with the nature of experience and knowledge and the relation between these. It involves an attempt to understand the condition of being in and experiencing the world while also addressing our awareness and interpretations of this condition. The concept of phenomenology has been imported into anthropology to refer to feeling and perceiving the world and to indicate a focus on sensate experience and the existential condition of being in a body.[7] Some use phenomenology to describe an effort to represent experience-in-itself in ethnography, prioritizing direct, subjective (though not necessarily embodied) experience over theory and interpretation.[8] I use the term here to refer to how one experiences—at the levels of consciousness, mind, body and other media—being in and living in the world, yet I also assert that there is not a single, universal phenomenology but rather multiple phenomenologies, multiple culturally and historically shaped ways of assembling and prioritizing the modes of experience through which people interact with the world.[9]

My assertion about the diversity of phenomenological orientations resembles Farquhar's 2002 claim that there is no single *a priori* state of embodiment, which she demonstrates by revealing how embodiment (embodied, aesthetic engagement with the world) changed from Maoist to post-socialist China in people's relations to food, sexuality, medicine and other realms of consumption and practice. Farquhar focuses on the body while her ethnographic analysis hints at a wider realm of aspects of the person that might help us theorize experience and how it changes historically. For example, she discusses those who delight in the emergence of the individual and interiorized self while also examining the development of an indulgence in the aesthetics of food and the sexualization of popular culture and everyday life in post-Maoist China. Similarly, I suggest that we need to consider the whole person as it is constructed at different times and in different places. Also, just as Farquhar suggests there are universal aspects of bodily desire, I assume that phenomenological orientations also contain within them truths of human experience that to some degree transcend time and place, but I propose that these are differently parsed and reconfigured in different localities. For example, all humans inhabit bodies—that is, embodiment is a universal existential condition in some sense—but many in India, including both lay thinkers and seasoned philosophers, feel that *ātman*, the intangible, true self, is the enduring, stable center of the human person and the state or position from which the person perceives the world. Some Indian thinkers also say that one should develop an awareness of the contingent and ephemeral nature of the body. In other words, Indian philosophy, both lay and professional, challenges Merleau-Ponty and much contemporary academic research that considers the body to be the existential ground of human experience. We should also remind ourselves that like Europe and the United States, India produces literate, phenomenological thinkers. For every Husserl, Heidegger and Dewey, there is a Śankara, Praśastapāda and Aurobindo, and these philosophers have had a role in shaping how people in India, and in other places where people are in dialogue with Indian thought, experience the world.

Furthermore, just as Farquhar shows how embodiment and people's engagements with aesthetics responded to government policies in China (for example, characterizing gastronomic pleasures as bourgeois indulgences), we will see how state policies and contemporary social processes in Kerala, such as the extension of facilities for and knowledge about allopathic and ayurvedic health care and the state's literacy efforts, have affected people's phenomenological engagements.

A phenomenological orientation is a guide to bodily, emotional, mental and other dispositions. It is a way of dividing up experience, leading a person to attend to and prioritize particular aspects of the body, the self, the person. My definition, however, is bound to the English language terminology and the phenomenological orientation that underlies labels such as "body," "mind" or "self." Essentially, the categories "body," "mind" and "self" as well as other aspects of the person in various cultural contexts are not anticipated by our academic analyses of experience and embodiment. For example, categories such as *bōdham* (roughly "consciousness") or *ātman* (a true, higher "self") are somewhat distinct from the "consciousness" or "self" of Western, intellectual parlance, and the relations between these categories of the person are culturally, and historically, shaped. *Ātman* and *bōdham* are distinct from *manas* (which itself is a more mechanical, cognitive "mind" than what is depicted by the English term), for example, and, according to philosophical writings, *ātman* has no specifiable characteristics. Although a phenomenological disposition mediates our experience and our relation to the world, I do not claim that a particular phenomenological orientation is necessarily all-determining, blocking the possibility of the immediacy of experience. Experience is shaped by our contacts and encounters with the world, and our phenomenological orientations train us how to organize and prioritize these contacts. We will see how people in Kerala are especially concerned about various states of "consciousness" and *ātman* as they encounter adverse life events, struggle with illness and navigate the variety of therapeutic options that are available in South India.

Aesthetic Experience in Healing

The experience of people undergoing treatment for psychopathology in Kerala affirms Laderman and Roseman's position that "if healing is to be effective or successful, the senses must be engaged" (1996: 4), but compels us to expand upon this insight. Researchers have analyzed the aesthetics of healing but have not compared the aesthetics of different medical systems or examined the aesthetic experience of biomedical treatment.[10] Thus, analyses of the aesthetics of healing do not explicitly recognize that the sensory engagements they explore are often agreeable or pleasurable experiences and thus do not fully reveal the benefits of this experience. Put more simply, it has been overlooked that a therapy that feels good might have some advantages over a therapy that is more painful or abrasive, especially for problems of mental illness.

Robert Desjarlais (1992) makes an important link between aesthetics and embodied experience in his analysis of healing in Nepal, explaining that Sherpa shamans make an ill person feel better through sensory, aesthetic engagement with the body: "Meme [a shaman] changes how a body feels by altering what it feels. His cacophony of music, taste, sight, touch, and kinesthesia activates a patient's senses. This activation has the potential to 'wake' a person, alter the sensory grounds of a spiritless body, and change how a body feels" (206). Desjarlais' analysis of Sherpa shamanism alerts us to the visceral experience of the shamanic healing process, but it would be intriguing to learn how this experience compares to the visceral experience of a biomedical hospital. Desjarlais explains that there is an allopathic medical facility available in the area where he did research, but it is a general clinic, not a psychiatric facility (163). People experiencing "soul loss" who were treated by a shaman did not visit this clinic for their problems. If allopathic psychiatric facilities were available, as there are in Kerala, they would likely claim to heal things like soul loss, which they would call by another name, and would constitute an alternative therapy.

Conducting research in Kerala, in which the institutionalization of multiple medical systems makes a diversity of treatment for mental illness widely available, I could compare the aesthetic experiences of patients in different therapies, including biomedicine. This allows me to bring attention to what one might call the positive and negative aesthetics of healing to more fully understand the significance of aesthetic engagements in the healing process.

Patient experiences with various treatments—such as ayurvedic mudpacks, allopathic electroconvulsive therapy and healing through singing and prayer—not only engage the senses. They engage the senses in both pleasant and adverse ways. There is no ideal term to designate this variety of sensorial engagements, but they can be described in terms of the relative presence and absence of "pleasantness." The term "pleasant" has limitations, however, and thus I will define how I am using this word. I use "pleasant" to indicate not only a positive sensory reaction but, in some contexts, engagement on the nontangible, "spiritual" level. "Pleasant" appropriately describes many patients' experiences in therapy, such as experiences in ayurvedic psychiatric procedures that patients say gave them a "cooling" effect, a local idiom for a pleasant physical sensation that has connotations of mental balance, or experiences living among the music, smells, color and scenic architecture of a Hindu temple. However, "pleasant" is at times too strong a term to indicate a healing process that is simply less abrasive than another form of treatment. For example, patients did not claim to like the purgatives or *ghee* some were given as part of ayurvedic treatment, but they were more averse to the electroconvulsive therapy they received during allopathic therapy. At other times, "pleasant" is too mundane a term to describe the more exalted changes some patients report in undergoing healing.

The observation offered earlier by Ajit that ayurveda can help one attain "another level" of health and pursue a "supreme aim" in life problematizes the notion of health as a simple remediation of symptoms and a return to functionality. While remediation of symptoms is a basic goal of therapeutic practices, some therapies also aim at instilling or increasing one's state of well-being, a state that is more enhanced, more vibrant than a simple return to a pre-illness or "baseline" state. Farquhar (1994) says that patients of Chinese medicine in China often expect to achieve a positive and active sense of health as a result of therapy: "It is often the case that neither patient nor doctor is satisfied with clinical work if all it achieves is a disappearance of symptoms. They are working with a language that can articulate a highly nuanced, positive, good health, and their goals are high" (482). Based on an analysis of ayurvedic texts, Alter (1999) likewise emphasizes that one of the goals of ayurveda is the continued pursuit of increasing good health—or "heaps of health" as he puts it. These are not just "exotic" ideals attributed to Chinese and ayurvedic medicine. A similar definition of "health" was once put forth by the World Health Organization.[11] Ajit feels such ideals of health are eroding, and he laments that "this is the level at which we maintain our health" referring to peoples' compulsions to find a quick fix for their problems so that they can return to work or school.

Along with these exalted goals of therapy are the more common, modest results of treatment that are not captured by the usual understandings of curing or healing. Thus people struggling with mental problems in Kerala talk of achieving *māram* ("change"), *bōdham* ("improvement") and *abhivriddhi* ("prosperity") through therapy. The attention to the process of therapy also makes us aware of ways of approaching time and teleology in therapy that also complicate the ideals of curing. For example, some people with chronic, recurring problems have found ways not of curing or healing, but of coping or living with their problems by residing in the aesthetically engaging environment of a temple, mosque or church. These people have been unable to rid themselves of their mental afflictions, but they have found a way of improving the quality of their experience as a person living with mental problems by choosing to reside in the aesthetically engaging setting of a religious center rather than pursue healing in the sterility or aesthetic adversity of a hospital environment.

This study also hopes to revive medical anthropology's concern with medical pluralism. This feature of the world of healing, which is indeed the norm of medical environments around the globe, was the focus of research going back to some of the earliest investigations in the field of medical anthropology, yet this topic has waned as a central concern in recent decades. Certainly numerous contemporary studies in medical anthropology continue to be set in medically plural environments, and the insights of some of these earlier works have been canonized in reviews of the field of medical anthropology (for example, Baer, Singer and Susser 2004). Nevertheless, the fact that most people in the world have the opportunity to "shop around" and compare medical systems could be more central to our analyses. Early studies of medical pluralism looked at how people navigate multiple healing systems, focusing on decision-making and cognitive, rather than experiential, orientations (Romanucci-Ross 1969, Janzen 1978, Young 1981). Later work looked at how people's interactions with multiple healing systems relates to socioeconomic change and social relations (Mullings 1984, Crandon-Malamud 1993), concerns about morality (Brodwin 1996), and, in my own earlier work, how medically pluralistic environments enable people suffering psychopathology to find a healing system that fits their personality and identity (Halliburton 2004). But the ability to compare medical systems also leads to insights into the aesthetic experience of healing and offers novel understandings of health and curing. By investigating these topics, this study reminds us of the fundamental importance of attending to the insights and experiences people develop from living in environments where multiple healing systems are widely available.

Kerala, "God's Own Country"

Looking out the window of a plane descending toward the airport in Trivandrum,[12] the capital city of the south Indian state of Kerala, I could see only a few buildings peeking above the thick growth of trees. It was impossible for me to discern a city of one million. Stretching along the Malabar coast of southern India, Kerala is in many ways a lush, tropical paradise, overgrown with coconut trees and blessed with beautiful beaches, but it is also one of the most densely populated states in one of the most densely populated countries in the world. Promoted as "God's Own Country" by the state tourist development board, Kerala has lured tourists to its backwater boat tours and ecotourist resorts that often feature "new-age" style reinventions of local medical practices, such as "ayurvedic massage." But this image belies the stressful modern, urban reality that commingles with tropical scenery in much of the state.

Like the tourists who sought "ayurvedic massage," I saw India as a possible source of novel medical insights, but I wanted to delve beyond the superficial and suspiciously neat depictions of ayurveda and other healing practices offered by much of the media in India and the West. I had come to Kerala to learn about the methods used for treating mental illness and the experience of people who undergo these treatments. Kerala is an ideal setting to examine these issues since the state has several elaborated, institutionalized forms of treatment for psychopathology that are broadly available. The comparative perspective brought by patients who use these therapies provides important insights into the nature of "mental" illness, the process of healing, and the character of mind, body, self relations that are not apparent in settings that are dominated by one system of healing.

Some in Kerala back the state tourism department's promotion of the state as "God's Own Country," an assertion about the lush physical beauty and ritual color of the state, while others see this as pretentious. Kerala is certainly colorful and alluring, but it is also crowded, stressful and afflicted by social problems that persist along with impressive achievements in education, health and social justice. What many Malayalis say about Kerala is that it is like Bengal, which is located at the other end of India, with several languages and cultures in between. Malayalis and Bengalis love seafood, eat a lot of coconut and enjoy soccer, while most Indians are solely cricket devotees. Malayalis also claim that their culture has produced significant figures in literature and film, and like the state of West Bengal, Kerala has repeatedly elected communist governments.

People in Kerala hold up their food as particularly emblematic of their identity. The rhetorical equivalent of "How are you?" when people meet in

KERALA

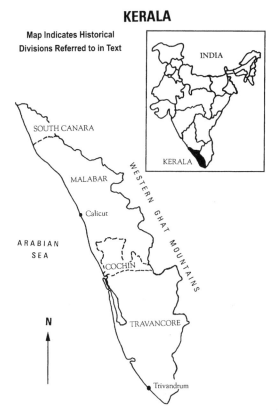

Map Indicates Historical
Divisions Referred to in Text

Map 1. Map of Kerala showing key research locations with names in Malayalam and English.

Map originally appeared in Richard W. Franke and Barbara Chasin *Kerala: Radical Reform as Development in an Indian State—Second Edition* Oakland, CA: Food First Books (1994). Reprinted by permission.

the afternoon in Kerala is "Have you had your lunch?" The taste for seafood and coconut may resemble Bengal, but Kerala cuisine is closer to that of neighboring Tamil Nadu: rice-based meals with numerous vegetable dishes flavored with mustard seeds, coconut and curry leaves and dosas (which are like sourdough crepes) along with other fried and steamed treats for breakfast and snacks. Food is frequently a topic of conversation in Kerala, and manifestations of mental problems I observed among patients at healing centers include refusing to eat, thinking food has been poisoned, and—as people prefer to mix, knead and eat the food on their plates with their hands—kneading food with one's hands for a long time before eating.

It is useful to think of the states of India as analogous to the countries of Europe. The borders of Indian states are generally determined on a linguistic basis, which often corresponds to significant cultural and historical distinctions, and as is the case with Europe, there is no language that the majority of people in India speak. The international borders between India and its neighbors Pakistan and Bangladesh reveal the ironies and contradictions of the contemporary nation-state. While border patrol personnel who speak the same language and eat the same food face each other from both sides of the India-Pakistan border, people in far-flung regions within India, such as Kashmir, Kerala and Nagaland can struggle to find much that they have in common. As one crosses the border from Kerala to its northern neighbor, Karnataka or its eastern neighbor, Tamil Nadu, one sees changes, sometimes abrupt, in language and culture. Just as someone familiar with Europe would not expect comments about social and cultural issues in Spain to be also true for, say, Finland, so one should not expect comments about life in Kerala to apply necessarily to practices in, say, Gujarat or Kashmir. Having emphasized the internal diversity of India, it is important to acknowledge that there are ideologies and practices that transcend regional and state identities. While this observation has unfortunately been used to disenfranchise non-Hindu citizens, many in India note that the practice of Hinduism extends to almost all regions of the nation while Sanskritic philosophy and literature has spread through, and plays a symbolically significant role in, much of the country—and, I will argue later, affects people's phenonemological orientation to experience in Kerala.

The natural fertility of the region, the availability of rice, spices and fruit, and an accessible location on the trade circuits of the Arabian Sea has attracted settlers and traders to the Malabar Coast for thousands of years, but currently resources are strained by Kerala's large population. Coconut trees are ubiquitous, yet there is a coconut shortage. The state is covered with rice paddy, but Kerala must import rice from neighboring Tamil Nadu to feed itself. The region has one of the highest rates of rainfall in the world, but there is often a shortage of water and rationing of hydroelectric power. Agriculture continues to be an important part of Kerala's economy, and the region continues to be enmeshed in overseas trade. Indeed, the so-called global economy is nothing new to this area although its specific features change. Whereas entrepreneurs once came to this part of the Malabar Coast from the Middle East and China to expand their trade networks and increase their wealth, today many Malayalis flock to the Persian Gulf countries in search of economic opportunity, with mixed success. Several of the mentally distressed Gulf migrants I spoke to attributed the onset of their problems to their experiences as migrants. Having traveled to Abu Dhabi or Dubai with the pressure of knowing that a good portion of the family wealth has been invested in an air ticket and visa, many migrants find that they are unable to make as much money as they had hoped to earn, and some, betrayed by their handlers who do not provide the employment they promised, have to return home broke, their families in worse financial shape than when they left. Some migrants who did find steady employment, usually in construction or other manual labor, relate the onset of their mental troubles to extreme homesickness, to not being able to handle the emotional strain of being separated from their families for long periods, although their mental problems persisted after moving back to Kerala.

The religious life of Kerala today reveals the long-term and ongoing connections of this part of the Indian subcontinent with far flung regions of the world. The majority of people of the Malabar coast consider themselves "Hindu," which in most of India is a mix of local practices and prestigious, brahmanical elements that are linked to classic Sanskrit texts. The southern Indian coast has seen numerous religious movements pass through, some of which, such as Christianity and Islam, stayed and some of which, including Jainism and Buddhism, gradually disappeared. In the first few centuries B.C.E., a community of Jews made their way from the Middle East to Cochin on the Malabar coast followed in the first century C. E. by a group of Christians who, according to one story, set out for southern India in an effort to inform the Cochin Jews that their Messiah had come. Islam made its way to South India in the eighth century brought by traders crossing the Arabian Sea, some of whom married local women and settled on the Malabar Coast. While today Kerala is approximately 60 percent Hindu, 20 percent Muslim and 20 percent Christian, and thus one of the most religiously diverse states in India, this part of the country has not seen the kind of violence that has erupted between religious communities in other places such as Mumbai, Ayodhya and Gujarat. Religious divisions do enter party politics and certain conflicts, but *Hindutva,* the Hindu fundamentalist political project that is at the center of controversies in Maharashtra, Gujarat and much of north India, has not had a strong presence in Kerala.[13]

Since 1956 when the princely state of Travancore was merged with the former British colonial territories of Cochin and Malabar to create the state of Kerala, the state government has been controlled mostly by communist parties, although coalitions led by the Congress Party have also seen several terms in office. Kerala's communist parties and grassroots social movements played significant roles in making quality health care and education broadly available in the state, and land reform and literacy movements brought a measure of socioeconomic equality to Kerala society.[14] Malayalis like to point to the fact that Kerala has the highest literacy rate in India, and they often add that this is one indication that Malayalis are, as they see it, more "educated" and "sophisticated" than people in other parts of the country. Kerala is anthropologically famous as the home of the once-polyandrous Nayar caste, although more recently investigators have been intrigued by the policies of the state's communist governments and Kerala's impressive "quality of life" indicators.[15] With a per capita income less than India's national average, Kerala's achievement of a literacy rate over 90 percent and life expectancy and infant mortality rates that are close to that of wealthy nations have turned the head of many socio-economic development specialists.[16]

P. Govinda Pillai, a member of the Communist Party of India (Marxist) and editor of the Malayalam political journal *Deshabhimani*, claims that communist government and social reform movements emerged from anti-caste struggles of the nineteenth century. He asserts that for a long period Kerala was marked by an extremely rigid and oppressive caste system, which eventually spurred low-caste leaders, such as Sree Narayana Guru (who is said to have influenced Mahatma Gandhi to oppose the caste system as part of his social reform agenda), to mount popular anti-caste struggles. That is, the inequities and excesses of the caste system, which were particularly pronounced in Kerala, impelled people at the bottom rungs of society to rebel.[17] Communism was later adopted as an ideology that complemented this social reform movement. And, as Malayalis like to remind people, Kerala's communist governments have always been democratically elected. They have also occasionally been democratically replaced by the Congress Party. Despite these impressive achievements, people in Kerala have struggled with high unemployment, which has resulted in heavy migration to Persian Gulf countries, and high underemployment, which appears to be linked to the state's high suicide rate.[18]

Malayalam, a Dravidian language related to Tamil, is the official language of the state of Kerala, and over 90 percent of the population speaks, reads and writes in Malayalam.[19] With 30 million speakers, Malayalam is only the eighth largest Indian language, but Kerala's high literacy rate makes it one of India's most significant literary languages.[20] Although the current level of literacy is partly due to late-twentieth-century grassroots and government efforts, literacy in Kerala is more than a project of modern political movements. Kathleen Gough explained that this was the most literate region in India during what she calls the "traditional" period of Kerala history (during the mid-fifteenth to the mid-eighteenth century, before the region fell under the hegemony of the British and the Mysorean empires). Gough shows that each sector of Kerala society had some reason for becoming literate: high agricultural productivity resulting from the region's heavy rainfall enabled a significant portion of the population to develop as literate specialists; the Brahmins brought their Sanskritic literacy from the North; the matrilineal Nayar caste became literate in their native Malayalam through their own teachers and most Nayar women learned to read; the Christians, Muslims and Jews were involved in trade and practiced religions that emphasized learning a sacred text (Gough 1968: 133, 151).

Kerala's literacy rate plays a role in shaping the world of illness and healing. As we will see later, people in Kerala learn about treatment options via newspapers and magazines. These same media sources disseminate popular and professional Western-style psychiatric discourse, which appears in patients' descriptions of their inner states in the form of English idioms such as "stress" and "depression." These idioms and discourses may in turn affect how patients experience their illnesses.

The Problem with Saying "Thank You" and Other Features of the Social Self in India

When I first arrived in Kerala I stayed with relatives of a friend from the United States who is originally from India. Based on American assumptions about hospitality, I had planned to stay with this family only a few days until I found my own place—after all, I thought, I only know their niece. This family, however, had assumed I would stay the whole year, and they were surprised and disappointed to discover that I wanted to find my own housing—after all, they figured, I know their niece. I explained that I had to move for my work, that living with them was enjoyably distracting and I was not getting enough done. Yet I quickly found that in Trivandrum, a city of one million people, there were very few realtors or agencies who advertised or rented places to individuals. If one needs a place to rent, one relies on word of mouth, one uses one's social network. I eventually learned—through friends and contacts, of course—of a person who finds places for rare individuals like myself who look for a place on their own.

I visited this realtor with the uncle of the family I was staying with. When we arrived at the realtor's office, the uncle spoke for me, telling the realtor what I wanted and responding for me as to whether a place was worth seeing—I, meanwhile, repeatedly tried and failed to gain an entree into the conversation to speak for myself. In the end, I did not choose any of the apartments shown by this realtor, and returning to the world of social connections, I ended up renting an addition in the house of a friend, a clinical psychologist whose insights on health and healing are occasionally cited in this study.

I tried to thank this family for their support, but that felt awkward, as I sensed this would be essentially a distancing gesture. The Malayalam word that translates as "thank you" (*nani*) is only used on formal or extraordinary occasions, as when addressing an audience or a judge in a courtroom, and not on a routine basis. It was hard for me to understand why people did not say *nani* until I asked myself why we say "thank you" in English. I realized that saying "thank you" was a way to symbolically give back what someone had given you, to even the balance so that people could go back to being autonomous individuals. "Thank you" is, among other things, a counterprestation so that one does not feel indebted or overly connected.[21] This would be inappropriate in Kerala.

There is very little privacy in Kerala, and it is generally assumed that people do not want to be alone. While I was living in Trivandrum, a friend would sometimes visit me unannounced by finding his way through my open back door and appearing in my living room. My research assistant, Kavitha, told me that she looked forward to having people to talk to when she commuted home from Trivandrum on the train—something that is difficult to imagine among urban commuters in the United States. Being alone is sometimes even considered dangerous, and many spirit-possessed people I spoke to became possessed when alone. Conversations between patients and their psychiatrists could sometimes be overheard by other doctors and patients who were meeting nearby, and inpatients often stayed in large communal rooms. Some doctors, however, did sequester themselves to speak with patients, and patients who could afford it paid for "private" accommodation at hospitals, which is to say that they stayed in a room with only their accompanying family members or friends.

Throughout this analysis of the lives of patients and their problems, it is important to be aware of the socially embedded, relational orientation to the self that pervades much of people's experience in India, which also co-exists with realms of autonomy. Much has been written about the sociocentric or dividual self in South Asia. In contrast to the egocentric or individual self, which sees itself as an autonomous entity that is separate from society, the sociocentric self is only intelligible in social context.[22] As Vaidyanathan (1989) describes:

> An Indian thinks of himself as being a father, a son, a nephew, a pupil, and these are the only "identities" he ever has. An identity outside these relationships is almost inconceivable to him. It is very common in Indian households to hear a person referred to as "Rekha's mother" or as "Babu's father," and the people concerned don't feel diminished in the least by these self-abnegating nomenclatures. (151)

The socially dispersed self repeatedly asserted itself during my stays in India. In fact, as in Vaidyanathan's example, I use relational names to identify relatives of ill people, such as "Sreedevi's mother," as these were the identities they presented to me.

It would be wrong to draw an overly neat distinction between an egocentric West and a sociocentric India. There are ways in which individualism co-exists with interpersonal connections in South Asia and situations that reveal sociocentric behavior among North Americans.[23] However, the notion that a person is not only connected to but embedded in her social relationships, the difficulty in abstracting the self from its social context, is crucial to comprehending behavior, action and desire in South Asia. Basic practices of daily life underscore this: people who were ill went for therapy, and for interviews with my assistants and myself, accompanied by one or several family members who did most of the speaking; people who bring a newspaper on a train will expect it to be shared by their fellow travelers; everyday discourse in Malayalam features many ways of aggregating the speaker and listener through subjectless sentences or by use of the inclusive form of "we" (which includes the speaker and listener) in situations where English speakers would use "you" or "I."

The term "sociocentrism" used by many researchers is not ideal for this orientation as what it involves is not quite a "centrism," a convergence on a single point. This metaphor is more appropriate when one speaks of egocentrism where the individual self constitutes the primary focus. With the "sociocentric" self, it is the variety of social relationships and the constantly changing social context that are significant. One imagines a network of relations with other selves rather than a central subject. The orientation to self in India might thereby be better characterized as a socially dispersed or socially embedded self.

Patients arrive at treatment centers with one or more family members who usually consult the doctor along with the patient, and this is how patients presented themselves to me and my assistants for interviews. At first I thought I should try to speak to the patient alone to get a more accurate idea of their concerns, and I did so on occasion. This may have brought out issues that would otherwise not have emerged, but it also amounted to editing out culture to some degree, imagining the internal, private self to be more authentic. The manner in which people I spoke with presented themselves made me realize that my interlocutor was not just the person suffering the problem but a "therapy managing group" of family, friends and others who are connected to the patient.[24]

The socially dispersed self also appears inpatient narratives. In translating interviews, my assistants and I often had to invent a subject to render a sentence intelligible in English. The subject of the sentence is often omitted in everyday spoken Malayalam, but the situation is distinct from, for example, colloquial Bengali or Spanish, where the subject is omitted but can be inferred by the conjugation of the verb (for example, *fuimos* in Spanish means "we," not "they" or "she," "went"). In Malayalam, even when the subject is omitted, the verb has exactly the same conjugation for each person (for example, *pōyi* could be "I," "you," "they" or anyone else "went"). Sometimes the subject is clear from context, but often it is—deliberately, I would argue—ambiguous. In interviews with people suffering illness, it is often impossible to tell, for example, if it was the mother speaking for the ill daughter, or the daughter, or both, who felt relief after a particular experience.[25]

The socially dispersed self is further revealed in ayurvedic methods of psychological counseling where it is permissible to give advice to a patient. Advice is ideally avoided in Western psychological and allopathic psychiatric therapy, where it is considered crucial that the patient develop her own insights. However, the individualistic ideals of allopathic psychiatry are not always upheld in psychiatric practice in India. One allopathic psychiatrist in Kerala, who had practiced for a period at a university medical center in the United States, said that in psychiatric practice in India one must more actively engage the family in treatment, and explained that early on in his consultations in Kerala he tries to identify a family member he can use as an ally in implementing treatment.[26]

Although the socially dispersed self is a fundamental part of life in South Asia, some cultural practices in India are highly individualistic. In Hindu religious practice, for example, there is no congregational worship (as there is in Islam, Judaism or Christianity) although people gather for special rituals. Instead a person decides on her own how to make the rounds at a temple, which one often visits alone. Strains of Indian philosophy, such as Yoga and Vedānta, can be viewed as individualistic, as attempting to distinguish the true self, *ātman*, from any social or phenomenal attributes; however, one might say that *ātman* represents a *universal* true self as distinct from the particularistic authentic self celebrated in Western psychology and literature.

The Comparability of Forms of Illness

I was asked by a psychologist in Kerala how I would define and standardize the kinds of illness I was examining in my work in Kerala. How many schizophrenics or depressive patients would I have in my sample, or how would I know what illness someone who was being treated for possession was suffering from? I explained that I did not want to privilege the illness definitions of any one therapeutic system, and I would therefore use the patient's and his or her accompanying family members' descriptions of the problem as the standard definition that transcended the various therapeutic contexts I was examining.

Meanwhile, allopathic psychiatrists I discussed my work with, both in Kerala and in the United States, were concerned about whether I was comparing problems of similar severity in my research. When I said that some people reported their condition had improved after their stay at Beemapalli mosque, psychiatrists suggested that this was probably because there were no seriously psychotic people at Beemapalli. They suspected that the mentally afflicted people at the mosque were only mildly neurotic and thus easily treatable by suggestion. This was a valid concern, but ultimately it did not reflect the kinds of people who frequented Beemapalli. Many of the patient-devotees at the mosque would be, or already had been, diagnosed by allopathic psychiatrists as psychotic. Several exhibited symptoms such as hearing voices, outbursts of laughing, crying, or screaming, tearing off clothes, flat affect, disordered speech, and outbursts of violence, and several had previously been inpatients in allopathic psychiatric hospitals.

The concern voiced by these psychiatrists did, however, reflect the need to interview people with problems of varying severity to obtain a more complete picture of the experience of psychiatric healing in Kerala. Fortunately, most research sites had something like a distinction between inpatients and outpatients based on the severity of the patients' problems, and I worked to balance my interviews along these lines. Both the allopathic and ayurvedic healing centers had outpatient and inpatient facilities, and the religious healing sites had similar distinctions. Some patients visited Beemapalli mosque on occasion and then went home whereas others lived at the mosque. Some people with serious difficulties who were violent or who were believed by their accompanying family members to be at risk of running away were locked in cells behind bars.[27] After reviewing the patient interviews, I found that a substantial portion of interviewees in each of the three therapies had problems that would meet the definition of severe mental disorder used by the World Health Organization in international epidemiological studies of mental illness.[28]

A related issue is whether states of possession and illnesses as understood by allopathic psychiatry or ayurveda are comparable or whether an illness category used by one healing system can be translated into the terms of another system. Is spirit possession a form of dissociative disorder? Is the ayurvedic diagnosis *kaphotmada* understandable as a type of depression, or vice versa? The relations between different forms of affliction have been discussed and debated, but I think the differences between these types of distress are impossible to discern fully—we may never completely comprehend how the existential experience of being possessed compares to the experience of coping with dissociative disorder or schizophrenia.[29] However, these conditions are comparable from a more pragmatic perspective in that people go to different healers for what they see as essentially the same problem. Many people I interviewed had visited, for example, both a psychiatric clinic and a temple known for healing possession in trying to find relief from their illness. There may have been different opinions about the nature of the affliction, and patients may have experienced their problems differently—they may have paid more attention to different manifestations or symptoms with different healers. However, the patient and his or her family would see the affliction as basically a single problem, and they can relate its history, all the ups and downs, through different forms of therapy. When we asked patients and their caretakers which healers or healing systems they thought had the most accurate view of their problem—when we asked, for instance, whether they agreed more with the view of the psychiatrist or the temple priest regarding their affliction—their response usually revealed that they were not particularly interested in this issue. We often received what sounded like gratuitous responses, that they agreed with all perspectives, but in almost every case they emphasized that what they wanted most was to get some relief from their problem. They did not care what kind of healer they visited. They were willing to try anything until they found something that helped.

Research in Kerala

This study is based on three periods of fieldwork in Kerala. Preliminary research was conducted for three months in 1994, followed by one year of fieldwork, from January 1997 to January 1998, during which patient interviews were conducted. On subsequent trips in 1999, 2004 and 2005, I revisited research sites and spoke with healers I knew about issues I encountered during earlier fieldwork.

My assistants Biju, Kavitha and Benny and I interviewed 100 patients of ayurvedic, allopathic and religious therapies about their illness histories and their experiences with various therapies. Thirty-two patient-informants (22 male and 10 female) were undergoing ayurvedic therapy at the time of interview, 35 (21 male and 14 female) were using allopathy and 33 (18 male and 15 female) were undergoing therapy at a mosque, temple or church. Sixteen healers were formally interviewed for this project, and I informally discussed problems of illness and healing with several additional healers. Informal conversations with healers became a routine, almost daily, practice while I worked in Kerala. Whether speaking to students and physician-teachers at the

Trivandrum Ayurveda College after giving a lecture on medical anthropology or chatting with psychiatrists after interviews at the Trivandrum Medical College, I found myself in regular dialogue with healers regarding problems of psychopathology and healing.

I also observed healing methods employed by the three therapeutic systems I was examining, and I monitored public discourse on mental health by reviewing popular magazines, television shows and movies and by attending conferences and workshops on psychological topics. Research sites included a government-run ayurvedic psychiatric hospital, two private ayurvedic psychiatric practices, three allopathic psychiatric hospitals (two public and one private), one Hindu temple, one Muslim mosque and one Christian church.

Although I speak Malayalam well enough for everyday, routine conversations, I was not proficient enough to converse smoothly in the vernacular on complex, personal topics. Thus, for patient interviews I required the assistance of T. R. Bijumohan "Biju," who worked as a clerk at an ayurveda college, and Kavitha N. S. and Benny Varghese, who were both graduate students in psychology at universities in Kerala.

We conducted semi-structured and unstructured interviews with patients and the relatives who accompanied them. Semi-structured interviews focused on the patient's illness history, the current status and features of their illness, the reasons the patient and caretakers chose the therapies they used, their reasons for changing therapies, their experiences with different therapies, their views about the cause of the patient's problem and their own prognosis for the problem. (The semi-structured interviews utilized the questions reproduced in Appendix A.)[30] In unstructured interviews, patients and their families had more latitude to determine the course of the conversation and raise issues that may not have been addressed in the more structured interviews. However, accepted and polite conversational style in Malayalam did not allow us to proceed directly through the semi-structured questions, and thus conversations between the informants, my assistants and myself during these interviews addressed the prepared questions but also regularly diverged into other topics.

All but one of the 28 unstructured interviews conducted were recorded on tape and transcribed. Most of the 72 semi-structured interviews were recorded with handwritten notes, but 11 of these interviews were taped. Thus, I have verbatim transcripts for 38 out of the 100 patients interviewed. At least six months after the original interviews, we attempted to conduct follow-up interviews with as many patients as possible to learn of any change in the status of their illness and their healing experience. My assistants and I obtained follow-up information on 25 patients either by interview or by mail-returned questionnaire. Informants were given the option of returning a questionnaire because follow-up interviews were hard to arrange, especially since many informants did not have telephones and were no longer visiting the treatment center where we originally interviewed them. Also, some patients lived a great distance from Trivandrum, where Biju, Kavitha and I were based.

Although we interviewed a substantial number of women, circumstances led us to include more male informants. Because I and two of my assistants, Biju and Benny, were male, it was generally easier for us to interview men. Male informants probably felt more comfortable talking to us, and norms of public interactions between men and women, especially among strangers, made it occasionally difficult to approach women for interviews. It was easier to interview female informants with my assistant Kavitha, who is female. However, because of restrictions on women traveling and staying out late and the fact that Kavitha lived farther from our Trivandrum-area research sites, it was necessary to conduct more interviews with Biju. Benny lived in northern Kerala and assisted only with interviews at the Government Ayurveda Mental Hospital. The gender of the informant did not always correspond to the gender of the assistant who accompanied me. Sometimes I visited a research site with Biju or Kavitha, depending on who was available that day, and we chose people to interview based on who had time and was willing. There were thus several occasions when Biju or Benny and I interviewed female informants and Kavitha and I interviewed men.

The assistance of Biju, Kavitha and Benny was invaluable. They had an excellent, almost therapeutic, rapport with the patients we interviewed, and they raised important insights regarding the healing systems we examined and the lives of the people we spoke with.

This study considers the aesthetic quality of healing in a medically pluralistic environment through chapters that move from the more ethnographic to the more analytical. Chapter 2 ("Three Therapies of South India") depicts the three systems of healing that are the focus of this study. Ayurvedic medicine is presented in terms of the official, text-based theories of ayurveda as well as observations of actual practice in clinics and hospitals. I discuss specific methods for the treatment of psychopathology in ayurveda, and in doing so I build the groundwork for understanding the aesthetic experience of patients who undergo these treatments. Allopathic medicine is alleged to be highly standardized, and ideally it is practiced in the same manner in every part of the world. Although there is significant uniformity in allopathic medicine, this chapter highlights unique features of allopathic psychiatry as it is practiced in India, such as the major involvement of the family in treatment. Finally, the rituals and routines one undergoes for illness at Chottanikkara temple,

Beemapalli mosque and Vettucaud church are presented. These places of devotion and healing feature aesthetically engaging environments where ill people sing, pray, dance about and act out compulsive behaviors amidst music, pleasant smells and scenic outdoor settings.

Chapter 3 ("Lives and Problems") presents the world of health and healing in Kerala from the point of view of the people who use these therapies. The chapter centers around the narratives of six people who were seeking treatment for mental problems (two from each of the three main forms of therapy) and presents their accounts alongside commentary on issues that arise in interviews, thus eliciting stories of illness amidst common cultural tropes and everyday concerns and pressures, including marriage prospects, family conflicts, work, education and Persian Gulf migration.

In Chapter 4 ("Experiencing the World from Body to *Ātman*"), I continue the discussion of the mentalistic West/embodied Other dichotomy in studies of the body and embodiment. Next, through informant narratives and selections from Indian phenomenological writings, I present the phenomenological orientation people engage with in Kerala as a continuum of states of increasing intangibility that range from the body to the immaterial higher self or *ātman*—an orientation that is neither a case of living through the body nor an example of mind-body dualism. I also examine social and historical factors that may have shaped this phenomenological orientation while showing how this orientation interacts with the mind-body dualism that has spread as a result of the proliferation of allopathic medicine.

Chapter 5 ("Cooling Mudpacks: The Aesthetic Quality of Therapy") provides a fine-tuned analysis of the recurring theme of the aesthetic quality of therapy that arises throughout this work by comparing specific allopathic and ayurvedic psychiatric procedures and examining informants' reactions to treatments and medications. Describing their experiences of allopathic and ayurvedic psychiatry, many patients reported that they disliked the effects of some allopathic treatments, such as electroconvulsive therapy and injections of psychotropic drugs, and that they found ayurvedic therapies, such as *talapodichil* (applying a medicated mudpack to the head), to be at best more pleasant or at least less abrasive to undergo. This analysis also considers relations between these aesthetic experiences and the phenomenological orientation outlined in Chapter 4.

As another manifestation of this focus on the process of healing, testimonies are presented from people who gave up pursuing medically oriented therapies after years of trying to resolve a chronic problem and found a solution to their difficulties not in a cure but through living in an aesthetically engaging, therapeutic environment at a mosque, temple or church. Limitations of the concept of curing are thus examined along with idioms patients use to describe what is accomplished in healing that diverge from English-language, allopathically informed concepts of "health" and "cure."

The discussion moves from Chapter 5 to Chapter 6 by explaining that while many informants are attracted by how ayurvedic therapy feels, many use allopathy because it provides quick results. Ajit reveals himself as a fan of ayurveda, a believer in its high ideals, yet he confesses that many people choose allopathy because of the time and work pressure that he sees as symptomatic of contemporary, functional orientations to health: "If I have a fever, I must get better [literally: must get changed—*māranam*]. For what? To go to work the next day. [. . .] This is the level at which we maintain our health." Indeed, allopathy often provides quick effects so that the patient can return to work, school or the many other obligations people have, although some in Kerala claim this constitutes a temporary repair rather than an enduring transformation of health. Chapter 6 ("Conclusion: Pleasure, Health and Speed") thus explores relations between time, work and aesthetics, suggesting that people in Kerala are caught in a dilemma between time pressure and pleasure while also revisiting views of health as absence of illness, the presence of well-being and the possibility of constant improvement.

Notes

1. "Allopathy" will be the term most often used to refer to the medical system that is also known as "biomedicine," "Western medicine," "cosmopolitan medicine," or "modern medicine." As "allopathy" is a popular term for this medical practice in Kerala, it is appropriate for discussing this ethnographic context. In addition, "allopathy" best describes how biomedicine is characterized in India and in this study. The term refers to the treatment of illness by opposites, for example, by using toxic substances that will kill a disease pathogen. This method can involve attacking an illness and employing abrasive techniques. Finally, "biomedicine" is somewhat misleading in the context of this study since ayurvedic medicine is also based on an understanding of biology, one that both overlaps with and departs from biomedical views of biology.

2. Translated from Malayalam, although words in quotations occurred in English in the original. In other writings, I have used the diacritical markings from the *American Library Association-Library of Congress Romanization Tables: Transliteration Schemes for Non-Roman Scripts* for transliterating Malayalam terms. Although technically precise and useful from the point of view of an expert in Malayalam linguistics, I have noticed that more reviewers of my writing have been confused by this system than have been helped by it. In this study I use a more informal rendering of Malayalam into Roman characters that excludes diacritical marks other than the line that indicates long vowels (e.g., ō in *bōdham*, ā in *ātman*) and an ś that indicates a particular light "sh"

sound (distinguished from harder "sh" which is transcribed as "sh"). Thus, rather than use, for example, an apostrophe as required by the *Romanization Tables* to indicate a letter that resembles the English "y" sound, I use a "y" (for example, *chaitanyam* rather than *caitan'aṃ*), and I use "n" rather than "n" with additional markings to indicate dental and retroflex versions of consonants that resemble the English "n."

The system I use closely resembles methods of transliteration employed in Kerala in English-language newspapers, advertising and signage where most of the text is in English and occasional Malayalam terms are rendered in Roman letters. I feel this will make the text more readable for those who are not experts in Malayalam but may know other Indian languages—although it may disappoint linguists. Tamil speakers, for instance, should easily be able to spot cognates they are familiar with, while Malayalam speakers should recognize which form of a letter is used by its context. This system also has the advantage of making it possible to render Malayalam terms as well as Sanskrit words, which occur in discussions of ayurveda in the text, using the same system of diacritics. Juggling two systems of transliteration would make the text less readable and occasionally confusing.

3. In this study, I use variations on Nichter's 1981 phrase "idioms of distress" (for example, "illness idioms," "idioms for expressing distress") to refer to the various forms in which illness or suffering can be expressed. This term has the virtue of not specifying problems as illness or disease but instead pointing to the more basic distress that characterizes psychopathology, family problems, possession and other, indeterminate forms of suffering. I also adopt Kleinman, Das and Lock's (1997) focus on suffering because it emphasizes a fundamental feature of problems I am examining without medicalizing them. For example, rather than referring to spirit possession as a mental illness or a symptom of such illness, I consider both possession and mental illness to be idioms of distress or problems of social, psychological and spiritual suffering.

4. Lakoff and Johnson (1980, 1999), Scheper-Hughes and Lock (1987), Csordas (1990, 1994, 1999), Strathern (1996).

5. Kleinman (1980) and Marsella and White (1982) represent examples of this orientation.

6. Kleinman in his work on depression and the expression of pain in China informs us that, around the world, somatization is a more common form of expressing distress than psychologization and is particularly found in non-Western societies: "Psychologization is the result of the Western mode of modernization that now influences the elite of non-Western societies; somatization is the product of more traditional cultural orientations worldwide, including that of the more rural, the poorer, and the less-educated in the West" (1986: 56). Psychologization, Kleinman claims, is a phenomenon of the middle- and upper-class Western world that emerged after World War I (55–56).

    Although anthropologists and other researchers do not usually explicitly say that all non-Western peoples are somehow more embodied, when one looks at the corpus of research on the body one gets the impression that people outside the West are more likely to ground experience in the body or that their experience transcends mind-body dualism. Frustrated by biomedicine's need to see all suffering as "either wholly organic or wholly psychological in origin," Scheper-Hughes and Lock propose that medical anthropologists try to transcend the assumptions

of mind-body dualism (1987: 9). Although they do not directly claim that all
non-Western cultures are holistic or locate experience more firmly in the body,
this characterization emerges when they suggest that "[n]on-Western and non-
industrialized people are 'called upon to think the world with their bodies'," yet
"[b]y contrast, we [Westerners] live in a world in which the human shape of
things . . . is in retreat" (23). Likewise, Andrew Strathern's *Body Thoughts* (1996)
contains characterizations such as "many peoples around the world . . . in whose
own cultural concepts emotion and reason are closely linked" (8), wherein emotion and reason represent aspects of the body-mind distinction, and references to
cultures where "this [European] kind of hierarchical ranking of knowledge versus
emotion does not exist" (151). Women and marginalized populations in the West
meanwhile have also been portrayed as somewhat more embodied (for example,
Fishburn 1997, Gilbert 1997, Quashie 2004). Ethnographic work subsequent to
these important forays into our embodied condition has not yet discovered the
variegated, subversively messy reality that is inevitably encountered after someone initiates an exciting new paradigm.

    Let me clarify that there is a difference between Csordas' work (1990, 1993,
1994) on embodiment and contemporary anthropological studies that focus
on the body. Csordas, and the phenomenology of Merleau-Ponty that informs
Csordas, sees embodiment as a universal human condition, and he asks us to consider the actual, lived experience of being in the body or "being in the world." All
people experience the world from the perspective of being in a body, and obvi-
ously this applies to people in Kerala. But considering this existential condition
is distinct from focusing on and scrutinizing the body as an object of knowledge.
Csordas (1999) distinguishes the anthropology of the body, which considers the
body as an external object of analysis, from embodiment, which he says is a methodological standpoint, looking/experiencing from the point of view of being in
a body. Additionally, I argue that the term "embodiment" has been employed by
many researchers, not to identify the existential condition Csordas describes via
Merleau-Ponty, but as a synonym for the body or somatization. When I critique
studies of embodiment, it is this use of the term as a synonym for the body that
I am most concerned with.

    Although they do not offer their works explicitly as critiques of the mind-
ful Westerner/embodied non-Westerner dualism, Lawrence Cohen (1998) and
Robert Desjarlais (1997) provide examples of works that engage the body along
with other modes of experience without assuming an embodied Other. Those
who focus on social suffering also offer the potential for an anthropology that
does not overindulge the body and considers a diversity of experiential conditions
(Kleinman and Kleinman 1995, Kleinman, Das and Lock, eds. 1997). Social suffering includes the notion of illness, but is broader, taking into account the mental, bodily and indeterminate other expressions of distress that stem from social
pressure ranging from stress to "nerves" to political violence.

7. Csordas (1994), Desjarlais (1992) and Weiner (1997).
8. Geertz (1986), Bruner (1986), Wikan (1991) and Jackson (1996).
9. This is similar to Desjarlais' definition of experience, in his ethnography of a
     homeless community in Boston, as "a historically and culturally constituted pro-
     cess predicated on certain ways of being in the world" (1997: 13).
10. For example, Kapferer (1983), Roseman (1991), Desjarlais (1992) and Laderman
     and Roseman (1996).

11. The WHO in 1978 defined health not as an absence of illness but as a presence of a sense of well-being, but this definition does not appear in recent WHO reports (1978, 2007a, 2007b).

12. This city is also known by its official Malayalam name, "Thiruvananthapuram," although people continue to refer to it as "Trivandrum"when speaking in English. The English and Malayali names of Kerala's two other major cities are Cochin/ Kochi and Calicut/Kozhikode.

13. This sketch of Kerala history is compiled from Narayanan et al. (1976), Dale (1990) and Sreedhara Menon (1990). See also Ghosh (1992), who reconstructs the life of a twelfth-century Jewish Arab merchant who traded with and settled in this region of South India, and Osella and Osella (2000a, 2000b) on Persian Gulf migration and social mobility in Kerala.

14. Thomas Issac, Franke and Raghavan (1998: 17–21) and Parayil ed. (2000).

15. For analysis of the Nayar caste, see Gough (1959) and Mencher (1965).

16. In 1995–1997, life expectancy was 63 years for all of India, 70 years in Kerala, and 77 years in the United States; infant mortality was 65 per 1,000 for India, 13 per 1,000 in Kerala, and 7 per 1,000 in the U.S. Adult literacy in 1991 was 52% in India, 91% in Kerala and 96% in the U.S. (from Governments of Kerala and India and World Bank statistics compiled in Franke and Chasin 2000: 18). Franke and Chasin (1994) and others claim that literacy in Kerala has reached 99 to 100% since 1991, although the literacy rate among my informants was around 90%. See also Parayil ed. (2000) for analyses of socioeconomic development in Kerala.

17. Govinda Pillai (1999). Desai (2005) also links Kerala's social achievements to nineteenth-century welfare expansions in the princely states of Travancore and Cochin.

18. See Mathew (1997) on unemployment and Halliburton (1998) on suicide.

19. Prabodhachandran Nayar (1994).

20. Although Kerala has only 4% of India's population, one of Kerala's newspapers, *Malayala Manorama*, claims to have the largest readership of any paper in India due largely to high literacy.

21. Wilce explains that in Bengali the term that translates as "thank you"is also rarely used, and Bengalis have a "tendency to foreground relationality and background personal autonomy"(1998: 10) in their interactions.

22. See Marriott (1976), Dumont (1970[1966], 1986[1983]) and Shweder (1991).

23. Mines (1988), Ewing (1991), Wilce (1998: 34–43) and Kusserow (1999). See also Nabokov's attempt to reconcile the personal, subjective self and the socially oriented self that co-exist within the Tamil person (2000: 13–15).

24. "Therapy managing group"is the term Janzen (1978) uses in his study of medical pluralism in Zaire to refer to the network of family, friends and others who are involved in coping with a person's illness.

25. Although the form of the verb can reveal the subject in subjectless constructions in Bengali, Wilce (1998: 83) explains that some degree of subject ambiguity is maintained in illness narratives and other "troubles talk" in Bangladesh.

26. See also Nunley (1998) on the involvement of families in Indian psychiatry.

27. Allopathic hospitals had similar facilities for violent patients, but the Government Ayurveda Mental Hospital where I conducted research in 1997 did not have such facilities. They could treat people with serious psychopathologies if they were not very violent. However, when I returned to Kerala in 1999, I found that

the ayurvedic hospital had moved to a new, larger facility that featured cells for violent patients.

28. Halliburton (2004).
29. See Kehoe and Giletti (1981), Lewis (1983, 1989) and Bourguignon (1991) on the relation between possession and psychopathology.
30. Semi-structured interview questions direct the topic of discussion, but allow open-ended responses. We did not use structured interviews, which are usually employed in more quantitative research and require forced-choice responses.

2

⚜

THREE THERAPIES OF SOUTH INDIA

People who suffer from mental difficulties in India have many options in their quest for relief. They could go to a *mantravādan* who uses magic if their family feels sorcery or evil eye, which can be invoked by the jealousy of another, might have caused the mental distress. They could visit a psychiatric clinic and receive pills or an injection, which are seen by many in India as fast-acting but dangerous modern medical interventions. Occasionally they may also receive some counseling at the clinic. They could go to the local mosque where a saint is buried and which people of all faiths visit in the hope that the munificence of the saint and the auspiciousness of the setting might help them overcome their illness. They might visit an ayurvedic physician and come away with pills, which they have heard are slower acting but less dangerous, less prone to side effects than allopathic drugs. They could end up in an ayurvedic psychiatric hospital where they might be treated with orally administered medications, cooling "mudpacks" and medicated enemas. Or a person suffering illness and her family may try one of many esoteric healers they have heard about from friends or read about in the newspaper: perhaps the Catholic priest who combines psychotherapy and yoga or the Hindu *pandit* who mixes spiritual teaching with his own version of ayurveda can help them find some "change," as they say in Kerala.

Ayurveda, allopathy and religious healing are the three most common forms of therapy for mental illness, possession and related problems in Kerala and in much of India. Ayurveda is an institutionalized system of

41

medicine that developed in South Asia and employs medications, dietary pre-scriptions and other interventions to treat illness. Kerala features ayurvedic facilities and physicians who specialize in treating mental disorders, and it is the practices these institutions and individuals engage in that I refer to as "ayurvedic psychiatry." Allopathic medicine is alleged to be uniform in its practice around the world, and there is a lot of truth to this. However, it should come as no surprise to anyone familiar with ethnographic analyses of such modernist institutions and their claims to universality that there are some uniquely Indian or Keralite features of allopathic psychiatry. "Religious therapies" is a somewhat more reified category when compared to ayurveda and allopathy. The latter two healing systems have institutional histories and canons of knowledge and practice while the "religious therapies" considered here are, more precisely, three different therapies: one that is practiced at a Muslim mosque, another at a Hindu temple and the third at a Christian church. These therapies do share an emphasis on the role of the divine and a person's relation to the divine in healing illness, though they also have their particular methods for doing so. The religious therapies and the two medical practices also overlap in some ways. For example, ayurvedic psychiatric medi-cines are sometimes administered at Chottanikkara temple, and counseling at Vettucaud church resembles the psychotherapy offered by allopathic psych-ologists and psychiatrists.

Ayurvedic Psychiatry

Whereas many ayurvedic practitioners in India treat mental illness, or *unmāda rog*, simply as an aspect of their general practice, Kerala is notable for ayurvedic physicians who specialize in psychiatry and ayurvedic facilities that specialize in the treatment of mental disorders.[1]

Summarizing Ayurveda

I am going to go ahead and commit the sin of trying to summarize ayurveda to provide context for understanding the treatment of psychopathology in this medical system. When I explain the kind of research I conducted in India, people unfamiliar with ayurvedic medicine often ask me to briefly explain how ayurveda works. This question conveys an expectation that ayurveda can be reduced to easily summarizable ideas and principles. Perhaps this is how we tend to think about any unfamiliar medical system, but I am sure it would sound odd to ask the same question about biomedicine.

My response to requests to summarize ayurveda is to say that in order to learn ayurveda one has to go to an ayurvedic medical school for three years and then work as an apprentice for a period of time afterward—which is similar to what is required to become a practitioner of biomedicine, although one can also learn ayurveda outside an institutional setting. This best summarizes ayurveda because it says that it is vast and complex, that it takes years to acquire a working knowledge. When asked to summarize ayurveda, I also try to offer some qualified comparisons to allopathic medical practices.

Perhaps to one who is raised in a society in which biomedicine is dominant, other medicines (collectively labeled "alternative" in North America) are assumed to be more simple or reducible to neat, holistic concepts. "Alternative" medicines are often imagined to have something in common with one another, and labels attributed to these therapies, such as "holistic" or "herbal," may be inspired by a yearning for what is lacking in biomedicine. At the same time, "holistic" is not necessarily a misleading description of ayurveda. There is a set of theories in ayurveda that practitioners attempt to relate to practice. Ayurvedic physicians do take into account diet, lifestyle, medication, the time of year and the patient's psychological state in considering an illness and its treatment, but then so do allopathic doctors to some degree. The difference is that there is a greater diversity of factors that ayurvedic physicians ideally should consider, and ayurvedic physicians show a greater concern for the effects of environment, diet and lifestyle on the physical states of the body.

The label "herbal" is somewhat appropriate as ayurvedic medicines contain more "natural" ingredients in the sense that these are less processed, subject to fewer laboratory refinements than allopathic drugs. However, ayurvedic medicines are often manufactured in factories, and the ingredients used are not limited to "herbs." Ayurvedic pharmaceutical manufacturers use original plant materials, as well as minerals and animal products, that contain naturally occurring active ingredients while active ingredients in allopathic medicines are often artificially created or replicated in isolated chemical form in laboratories.

Another salient difference between allopathy and ayurveda is seen in each system's relation to its early, foundational medical texts. Whereas the medical writings of Hippocrates, Aristotle and Galen are no longer regularly invoked in contemporary allopathic research and practice, ayurvedic researchers and practitioners frequently dialogue with classic texts including *Caraka Saṃhitā* (composed between 1000 B.C.E. and 200 C.E.), *Suśruta Saṃhitā* (composed between the seventh century B.C.E. and 0 C.E.) and *Aṣṭāṅgahṛdayasaṃhitā* (sixth to seventh century C.E.).[2] These treatises, written by early physicians, describe principles and attributes of bodily function, explain specific treatments for specific afflictions, and provide epistemological and practical guidelines for the practice of medicine. Ayurvedic physicians and educators today frequently cite these *samhitās* as they explain the uses of particular treatments or discuss a case with a colleague. There is even some competitiveness in citing classic texts among specialists in ayurveda. A physician's ability to quote by memory extensive passages from classic texts in the original Sanskrit confers admiration from other physicians and students. The classical texts do not thoroughly reflect contemporary ayurvedic practice, however, and part of the art of ayurveda today involves reinterpreting classic texts in terms of contemporary contexts—by explaining for example that certain regimens described in a classic text might not be feasible given people's contemporary lifestyles or simply observing that a certain ingredient is substituted in a particular medicine because the ingredient mentioned in the classic text is no longer available.

Ayurvedic concepts and practices are also influenced by four schools of philosophy that were founded in the second and third centuries: *Nyāya, Vaiśesika, Sāmkhya,* and *Yoga.* These schools engage issues of epistemology, knowledge about the workings of the physical world, explanations of the origin of the universe, characteristics of the body, mind and consciousness and methods of logical reasoning.[3] *Nyāya* is a system of thought, logic and observation that is not unlike the epistemology that underlies Western scientific method. It is positivistic and makes claims such as, "Perception, inference, comparison and word (verbal testimony)—these are the means of right knowledge," and, "Perception is that knowledge which arises from the contact of a sense with its object, and which is determinate [well-defined], unnameable [not expressible in words], and non-erratic [unerring]."[4] The discourse of the *Nyāya Sutras* resembles Karl Popper's struggles to define the nature of positivism and objective perception, but *Nyāya* often transcends the Western, academic religious-secular dichotomy by describing things such as the character of the soul or true self through syllogisms and other positivistic arguments.

Ayurveda is also informed by recent books, journals and research papers. Although *Caraka* and *Suśruta* are still routinely invoked, ayurvedic specialists engage in ongoing research and are influenced by practices of allopathic medicine, features of which are embraced or opposed by various ayurvedic practitioners. For their thesis requirements, students at the Ayurveda College in Trivandrum conduct clinical studies of new ayurvedic methods of treatment and attempt to clarify and test classic concepts through contemporary scientific research methods (that is, Western/international/biomedical methods, using statistical analyses and control groups) while *Aryavaidyan* and other journals publish the results of contemporary clinical research in ayurveda. Some ayurvedic physicians explained to me that ayurveda is translatable to

Western-style scientific and allopathic terms and asserted that the two medical systems are not radically different from one another. Others maintain that ayurveda is distinct, and they are critical of the practice of continually updating research and treatment methods. They believe that such attempts to update ayurveda simply imitate the epistemology and methods of allopathy, which is constantly abandoning earlier techniques and concepts, indicating, in their eyes, a lack of reliable, tried-and-true practices.

Leslie (1992) and Langford (2002) have likewise observed a distinction between syncretists and purists in ayurveda. Leslie (1992) suggested that syncretism among medical systems is a feature of South Asian cultures, yet purists in India advocate through professional organizations that ayurveda should remain distinct. The purist position is partly a reaction to biomedicine shaped in the context of postcolonial identity struggles that emerge with developmentalist discourses. In fact, the emphasis on gentle and non-abrasive medical procedures that will be considered in Chapter 5 may have developed in response to allopathic practitioners' control over performing more invasive, violent procedures (such as surgery) that were once also the province of ayurvedic physicians (Zimmermann 1992). Langford (2002) explains that the term "ayurveda" designates a diversity of practices. Ayurveda is taught in colleges that resemble biomedical schools in their institutional structure, while physicians who work and teach in these institutions, claiming an authoritative text-based ayurvedic knowledge, are haunted by the claims to authenticity of *vaidyans* (a more "traditional" term for an ayurvedic practitioner) who have been trained outside of academic institutions through the guru-disciple method (188–230).

The awareness of colonial and postcolonial processes of imitation, resistance and competition can make a "real" ayurveda appear elusive or highly contingent. It is important to recognize that the diversity of styles and claims to authenticity demonstrate that ayurveda is not a uniform or timeless system. However, it is possible to identify features of ayurvedic medical practice, or at least of contemporary ayurvedic practices. The canonization of key texts indicates some degree of character or stability or at least an axis of issues that re-emerge in ayurveda, even if these are reinterpreted in different periods. Moreover, one can speak of an ayurvedic system in terms of how it diverges from, and parallels, other healing systems such as allopathy or religious therapies. Trying to draw the boundaries around "ayurveda" as a medical system is an elusive process that is subject on the one hand to essentialization and reification and on the other hand to a process of deconstruction that can make it appear that ayurveda has no definable characteristics. My solution to this dilemma in the present work is to qualify my description of features of ayurvedic ideals and practices by emphasizing that what I describe are dimensions of contemporary ayurvedic practice that have emerged, mostly but not exclusively, in institutional settings in South India. The contemporary practices are informed by classic texts interpreted in contemporary contexts and configured partially in relation to allopathic discourses and practices.

One of the first characteristics that is usually highlighted in descriptions of ayurveda is its knowledge[5] of three *dosas*—*vata* (often translated as "wind"), *pitta* ("bile") and *kapha* ("phlegm")—which underlie the functioning of the body and mind. *Dosa* is often translated as "humor," which, while no translation can be completely adequate, has the problem of invoking an image of substances flowing around the body. For many, the term "humor" calls to mind a quaint, outdated medical concept, a belief people had about substances that circulated in the body until anatomy revealed the truth of human physiology. *Dosas* are probably best seen as principles of relationship, or as Zimmermann (1995) suggests, mnemonic devices, ways of thinking about the body. Yet *dosas* should not be viewed as abstract. Although they cannot directly be seen in the way blood or other bodily substances can, they underlie and affect tangible characteristics of the body, as well as other substances of nature.[6] "Wind," "bile" and "phlegm" are common, but limited, translations for the *dosas*: *vata*, *pitta* and *kapha*. "Wind" is probably the best of these translations, but the meaning of *vata* is more precise if one can imagine, in addition to the notion of wind, the principle that is inherent in wind, in dryness and in motion. "Bile" is improved if one also adds the notion of fire or heat, and *kapha* features characteristics such as "coolness" and "slowness" in addition to "phlegm."

Ayurvedic texts also describe seven *dhātus*, or substances of the body: *rasa* (lymph, plasma), *rakta* (blood, or more specifically the colored agent of blood, something like hemoglobin), *māmsa* (muscle), *medas* (fat), *asthi* (bone and cartilage), *majja* (marrow), *śukra* (seed, reproductive substance).[7] In addition to *dosas* and *dhātus*, ayurvedic medical knowledge includes numerous other categories related to functions and processes of the body, mind and intellect, such as *gunas* (mental dispositions), *malas* (bodily waste products), *agnis* (transformative agents), and *srotas* (channels of circulation).

Disease can arise from vitiation of *dosas*—excessive or insufficient activity of one or more *dosas*—which can result from diet, behavior, environmental factors and other influences. Healing is effected by prescribing medications, diet and lifestyle changes designed to improve the activity of the *dosas*. Several books on ayurveda, especially those written for a popular audience interested in alternative health regimens in the United States, Europe and India, often describe ayurvedic therapy as restoring balance to the *dosas*. Alter's 1999 critique of the remedial bias in medical anthropology through his analysis of ayurvedic views of health, as well as my own observations on the limitations of the ideology of curing, suggest the return-to-balance metaphor may involve importing biomedical assumptions about curing as ridding of symptoms and restoring functionality. Another way to look at the goals of healing in ayurveda is to think of balance as an ideal state of health that one should strive for. As Alter suggests, people are not seen in ayurveda as normally in balance before illness and as having returned to a state of balance after treatment. Rather, each individual in her normal state, absent of any illness has a dominant *dosa*, or *dosas*, a certain body type or disposition. That is, people are usually not balanced, and in states of illness their *dosas* are even more greatly misaligned. Treatment, whether for a pathology or for health improvement, aims to correct the problematic *dosa(s)* and move the patient closer to a state of dosic balance. This continuum of experiences of incremental improvement toward an ideal state can be seen among patients in Kerala who talk of achieving states of healing that range from simple "change" (*māttam*) to positive transformation.

These conceptual features of ayurveda are described in texts and taught in colleges and to some degree inform the practices of ayurvedic physicians. However, it is difficult to explicitly see the theory of the *dosas* and other principles in everyday practice. Instead one often observes doctors simply prescribing medications to treat a particular patient's illness. If asked, some practitioners say they are unable to explain the *dosaic* principles involved in a therapy while others do offer connections to these principles.

The connection between practice and basic principles is more pronounced among physicians who practice a method of treatment that involves tailoring medications to individual patients' problems. Today ayurvedic medicines are processed in laboratories, packaged, and sold in pharmacies that are hard to distinguish from allopathic pharmacies. Both ayurvedic and allopathic pharmacies sell factory-made packages of pills, capsules and liquids, but some ayurvedic pharmacies also sell raw medicinal plant materials. This standardized, factory-based method of production differs from what is considered a "traditional" method of ayurvedic practice involving the mixing of ingredients to create medications that are specific to each patient's unique condition. Using the latter method, doctors combine their knowledge of ayurvedic conceptual principles and pharmacology to either mix together a medicine designed to treat a particular patient's constellation of symptoms or write a prescription tailored to a particular patient's problem in the form of a recipe that the patient's family prepares at home using raw plant materials obtained from an ayurvedic pharmacy.[8] This method continues to be used by some practitioners in Kerala, but appears to be changing in relation to changes in the ayurvedic drug industry, which has begun to standardize the production of pills and other medications, possibly to increase production and profitability or to conform to what allopathy has established as a normative style of producing medication. Kerala's large pharmaceutical manufacturer Arya Vaidya Sala started in 1902 as an attempt to standardize and legitimize ayurvedic pharmaceutical practices following the model of biomedical practices (Habib and Raina 2005: 75), and ayurvedic reseachers at a plant pharmacognosy center in Trivandrum are today working to further standardize ayurvedic medicines by developing ways to regulate the quantity of active ingredients in ayurvedic products.

The creation of tailor-made medications may be linked to the tendency in ayurveda to approach treatment not in terms of disease categories but in terms of specific patients with specific symptoms of distress. Although ayurvedic physicians use disease categories, they also employ a conceptual continuum that is informed by *dosas*, among other things, to explain particular constellations of symptoms in individual patients. For example, a person who visits an ayurvedic physician with complaints about stomach cramps and headache will not necessarily be identified as having a particular disease indicated by these symptoms. Instead he may be seen as a person with stomach cramps and headache, and those particular symptoms (and the excess or insufficiency of *dosas* that underlies them) will be treated. This orientation to treating individuals with symptoms may help explain the attention to the aesthetic quality of the process of treatment in ayurveda. Perhaps a greater emphasis on destroying pathogens (and the often-cited war metaphors that are invoked in this effort) enables allopathic treatments to focus more intently on the ideal of *curing* and employ more abrasive treatments—as will be discussed further in Chapter 5.

It should also be mentioned that ayurveda is not confined to South Asia, but has emerged in various parts of the world. There are ayurvedic healing centers in major U.S. and European cities, and ayurvedic medicines are sold in health food stores and pharmacies in many other countries. In the United States, Deepak Chopra has brought his version of ayurveda to popular audiences through the media, and the Body Shop as well as other body and skin care manufacturers feature products that claim to be ayurvedic. At an ayurvedic center in New Mexico, meanwhile, ayurvedic *panchakarma* therapy, which is administered to patients at the Government Ayurveda Mental Hospital in Kerala, is marketed as a spa treatment to New Age American consumers (Selby 2005: 121). The marketing of ayurveda abroad, and to a great degree in India as well, emphasizes holism, balance, nonviolence, use of natural products and vegetarianism. Zimmermann has described this trend as a commodification of ayurveda that has developed in relation to biomedicine due to "the current quest for gentleness in the competitive marketplace of alternative medical care" (1992: 218). Thus, the attention to the pleasantness of the process of treatment in ayurveda may have been shaped by competition with biomedicine and other therapeutic systems.

Theory and Treatment of Psychopathology

According to ayurveda and certain schools of philosophy in India, the person is made up of a physical, a subtle and a causal body. A person possesses *buddhi* (intelligence, intellect), *manas* (similar to mind), *indriyas* (sense organs), *ahamkāra* (a sense of self or individuality) and other attributes that constitute what might be considered one's "mental" make-up, although as will be seen later, the person is constituted by a continuum of states that range from the tangible to the intangible in which the mind is less tangible than *buddhi* but more tangible than the body. Mental illness can develop from vitiation of any or all of the three *dosas* or excess in the mental humors *rajas* and *tamas* due to excessive desire (for example, lust or covetousness) and repulsion (avoiding objects that cause pain).[9]

Rather than offer my own overview of elements of ayurvedic treatment of psychopathology, I will present descriptions of this specialty by three well-known Kerala ayurvedic psychiatric specialists, along with my observations of their practices. As mentioned earlier, Kerala is reputed for its ayurvedic psychiatric practices and features specialists who treat people with mental problems, while in most regions of India psychiatric therapy in ayurveda is usually handled by general practitioners. Ayurveda colleges do not offer specialized degrees in the treatment of psychopathology. A person who wishes to specialize in the ayurvedic treatment of mental disorders must obtain a general medical degree in ayurveda and then apprentice with a specialist such as Dr. Sundaran.

Dr. K. Sundaran is an ayurvedic physician and college lecturer who is well known and widely respected in the ayurvedic community in Kerala. When I first met him in 1994, he was a physician at the Government Ayurveda Mental Hospital (GAMH) in Kottakkal, a small city in northern Kerala that is the home of several ayurvedic institutions and research centers. Dr. Sundaran completed his basic ayurvedic training at Ayurveda College in Trivandrum in southern Kerala and then earned a graduate degree at Gujarat Ayurveda University in north India. Dr. Sundaran worked at the GAMH in Kottakkal from 1986 until 1994 when he went on deputation from his duties to teach in the Trivandrum Ayurveda College as Senior Lecturer in the Department of Basic Principles. While teaching in Trivandrum, Dr. Sundaran also saw patients, and his reputation as a healer drew clients from a great distance. Some patients took a nine-hour train journey from northern Kerala to consult with him, and some came from other states. When I last saw him in 2005, he had returned to the GAMH in Kottakkal and was also supervising student training for matriculates at the Kottakkal Ayurveda College.

In my first meeting with Dr. Sundaran in 1994 at the GAMH, I realize in retrospect, I essentially asked him to summarize the theory and practice of ayurvedic psychiatry for me, and rather than repudiate my naïve, overbroad request, he made a thorough attempt to answer it. The following depiction of the etiology and treatment of psychopathology is compiled from this and subsequent meetings with Dr. Sundaran. He began by describing personality formation, which is important for understanding the development of *unmada* (mental disorder). His explanation started at the earliest moments of development, outlining the six factors that contribute to personality formation in utero: (1) father's sperm, (2) mother's ovum, (3) the mother's diet while pregnant, (4) activities of the mother while pregnant, (5) particular characteristics of the uterus and (6) climate of the region where the birth occurs. At a later meeting, Dr. Sundaran added that the *dauhridaya*, or "two hearts," period in pregnancy contributes significantly to the development of personality. The "two hearts" refers to the fetal heart and the mother's heart, and it is suggested that the desires of the mother during this period are transferred to the child. Dr. Sundaran enumerated additional factors that affect the development of the personality after birth: (1) one's religion, (2) type of family or communal group, (3) place—such as topography or rural or urban residence, (4) environment—including climate, soil, nature of foods grown in the region, (5) age and (6) other details, such as education level, the character of one's friends and travel experiences. Thus, like anthropologists, ayurvedic psychiatrists emphasize social context in explaining the development of the individual personality.

Dr. Sundaran went on to explain that there are two basic types of *unmada*: those related to exacerbated *dosas*—excess or insufficiency of *vata*, *pitta* or *kapha* resulting in mental and somatic problems—and those related to personality disorders, which involve specific aberrant behaviors. Most patients at the Government Ayurveda Mental Hospital officially received *dosa*-related diagnoses including: *vatotmadam*, characterized by manic behavior, hyperactivity, running away from home and delusions; *pittotmadam*, which manifests in behaviors such as outbursts of anger, acts of violence, overeating and drinking excessive amounts of water; and *kaphotmadam*, wherein the patient is lethargic, gloomy and passive. Dr. Sundaran also explained that *graha* diagnoses, which are specific types of behavioral disorders ranging from megalomaniacal behavior to acting like particular animals, are rarely used and few specialists know how to diagnose these problems. Two additional diagnoses used by people treating psychopathology in ayurveda that do not fit into either the *dosa*-related or *graha* categories are *bhayam*, a state characterized by fear or a general phobia, and *vishadam*, which is akin to the allopathic category "depression" and is caused by external factors such as shock. *Vishadam* is similar to *kaphotmadam* except that *vishadam* can involve problems with anger, which are not characteristic of *kaphotmadam*.

The *dosa*-genic disorders can result from excessive desire, trauma, shock, dietary problems and other factors, and treatment involves taking medications, undergoing *snehapana* (drinking ghee to oleate the body and facilitate the removal of impurities), taking an oil bath, sweating, *panchakarma* (a two-week course of purification/detoxification therapy consisting of five steps: emesis, purgation, medicated enemas, non-medicated enemas and medicines taken through the nose) and talk therapy. Many ayurvedic psychiatric medications and therapeutic procedures, according to Dr. Sundaran, work on the *sringart-aga*, an area of the head about halfway between the forehead and the apex of the head. This is the point of convergence of four senses (taste, hearing, smell and sight) and is the center of mental activity in ayurveda.

Cooling the Mind at the Government Ayurveda Mental Hospital

Kerala's Government Ayurveda Mental Hospital is located in northern Kerala in Kottakkal, a town that is home to several other ayurvedic institutions including the Arya Vaidya Sala, an organization founded in 1902 by the *vaidyan* Vaidyarathnam P.S. Varier. The Arya Vaidya Sala currently operates a drug-manufacturing center, hospital, nursing home, botanical research garden and ayurveda college in Kottakkal. The Government Ayurveda Mental Hospital, founded in 1984 and funded by the Government of Kerala, is one of the few ayurvedic institutions in Kottakkal that does not operate under the auspices of the Arya Vaidya Sala organization.

The mental hospital is staffed by a director, two psychiatrist-physicians, four nurses and several other attendants. Just over twenty outpatients are seen every day, and at any time approximately eighteen inpatients (about 13 male, 5 female) are staying at the hospital. When I visited in 1999, the GAMH had moved from the old Malabar-style mansion in which it had been located to a larger, modern facility that holds fifty patients, and the size of the staff had increased.[10] Most of the following description is based on observations of the hospital at the old facility in 1994 and 1997. Treatment at the hospital is free for patients who earn less than Rs. 1,500 per year ($45 U.S., the average annual income in Kerala being close to $200 U.S. at the time). Patients earning more than this amount are required to make some contribution to their treatment on a sliding scale. Most of the patient contributions go toward the cost of medicines, which are becoming increasingly expensive.[11]

Patients are admitted to the hospital after an outpatient consultation or a period of outpatient treatment. These consultations involve ascertaining the patient's symptoms, assessing the patient's overall state of health, giving memory tests and trying to evaluate the patient's normal personality to determine to what degree the patient's behavior deviates from her normal state.

According to staff physician Dr. Abdu, the inpatient treatment process at the hospital lasts 45 days, and patients may repeat the course of treatment up to three times, depending on the severity of the problem. Upon arriving at the hospital, patients are given medicines for one week to relieve their symptoms after which they do *snehapana*, which involves drinking medicated ghee (clarified butter) every day for a week in amounts that increase by 60 ml per day. The purpose of *snehapana* is to lubricate the body, and during this time the patient is restricted to a diet of *kanji*, a mildly flavored rice soup. After resting for a day following *snehapana*, the patient is given oil baths and steam baths to induce sweating. The baths are administered over two days, after which patients begin the therapeutic procedure known as *panchakarma*. *Panchakarma* is described in the classic ayurvedic texts, although it is not often used today outside of Kerala.[12]

Panchakarma begins with a day of *vamana*, where a drug is given to induce vomiting, followed by *virechana*, in which a purgative is taken to empty the bowels. These steps plus the preliminary *snehapana* and sweating and later steps in *panchakarma*, remove "impure substances," from the body. Dr. Abdu explained: "The purpose of *snehapana* is lubrication of the body. . . . impure substances are lubricated by this treatment. Then by way of fomentation [sweating], these impure particles go to the alimentary canal. While in the alimentary canal, some will come to the nose and others to the stomach and intestines. The substances reaching the stomach are expelled by way of vomiting. For other substances, which leave through the intestine, we give purgative medicines."[13]

After the purgative treatment, *virechana*, and a day of rest, patients are once again given medicines for specific symptomatic relief through the remainder of their stay at the hospital. The next step in inpatient treatment at the GAMH is the application of enemas or *vasti*. *Snehavasti*, an unmedicated enema with oil, and *kashayavasti*, a medicated enema, are given alternating with days of rest for a total of four *snehavasti*s and three *kashayavasti*s over the course of seven days. *Panchakarma* therapy ends after a week of *nasya*, which involves steaming the head and administering medicine through the nose.

During the remaining two weeks in the hospital, patients undergo *picchu* and *talapodichil*. *Picchu* involves pouring medicated oil into two cloths that are tied around the top of a patient's head. The cloth is then left on the head for a period of time while the oil is absorbed through the skin. *Talapodichil* consists of applying a medicated gooseberry "mudpack"—a combination of gooseberry, buttermilk and other ingredients that looks like mud or wet clay—to the patient's head and tying it in place with a banana leaf. After 45 minutes, a *marma* halfway between the forehead and the top of the head is said to warm to a temperature of 40° C. *Marmas* are physiologically significant points on the body that are engaged in understanding the functioning of the body and the administration of some treatments, and this *marma* is considered an important locus of mental activity. At this time, the mud from the area around the *marma* is removed and replaced with fresh, cooler mud.

In observing administrations of *talapodichil*, I was struck that patients who were undergoing this therapy were in a good humor. They reported that the procedure provided a pleasant, cooling effect, and they joked about how the banana leaf looked. I thought it significant that the mood and atmosphere among patients undergoing *talapodichil* and other ayurvedic therapies described here contrasted with the seriousness and occasional trepidation I observed among patients undergoing allopathic inpatient procedures such as the administration of psychiatric medications and electroconvulsive therapy. Patients did not dread, and often appeared to enjoy, treatment at the GAMH although not all embraced the lengthy, austere regimen one had to undergo while in therapy—for example, not being able to eat meat or fish or smoke was a struggle for several male inpatients (many in Kerala say they cannot get through the day without their fish curry and I began to feel the same way after extended stays).

My understanding of the purpose of these procedures is that they calm and "cool" the patient, which has connotations of mental balance and a positive sensory effect, and remove impurities (it might be helpful to think of this as a removal of toxins) thereby making medicines and talk therapy more effective. The calming and cooling effect patients report is also therapeutic in and of itself, while the implications of the pleasantness of undergoing these procedures will be a topic of further scrutiny a little later.

Before continuing with further details about ayurvedic treatments, I should emphasize that many in India are concerned about biopiracy of local medical knowledge, the misappropriation of ayurvedic medical knowledge by researchers and producers who intend to develop commercial products based on this knowledge. *Botanical researchers and drug producers are required to consult India's Traditional Knowledge Digital Library (www.tkdl.res.in) to obtain official access to medical information and information on profit-sharing requirements for products that are produced based on ayurvedic knowledge.*

The medications given to patients at the GAMH are designed to treat their specific pathologies. Dr. Sundaran treats many of his outpatients with a powder made of the medicinal plant *sankapushpi* (Sanskritic name for *Clitoria ternata*), which he says provides "rejuvenative power for the brain."[14] *Sankapushpi* is also administered by some Muslim priests in Kerala to treat mental problems, according to Dr. Sundaran. Dr. Sundaran sometimes prescribes a variety of medicines, such as a mixture of *Asafoetida indica, Acorus calamus,* and *Barbarus aristata,* to be taken by outpatients as *dhumapana,* a method of administering medicine that involves rolling plant materials into a cigar that the patient smokes by inhaling through one nostril and exhaling through the mouth. While it is not possible here to provide a complete overview of ayurvedic psychopharmacoepia, a depiction of the medical regimen of two inpatients from the GAMH provides examples of the application of medications to particular problems of psychopathology. This information is reproduced verbatim from patient charts with my summaries of Dr. Sundaran's explanations of the purposes of some of these medicines added in brackets:

> Case #1: Reasons for admission: fear, lack of sleep, restlessness, overly anxious, angry, doubtful, sorrowful.

> Medicines: 1) Special powder [see below] 2) *avipatti* [purgative: a combination of ten drugs]—alternate days 3) *ashwagandharishtam* [improves general physical and mental health]—30 ml 2 × day 4) *kanjunyadiennu* [improves sleep in some people] on the head 5) *manassmitravadakam* [for general improvement of mental functions, but expensive as it contains gold—only prescribed if patient can afford it] tablets—1 per day. After 7 days, give *snehapana* with *panchagavyaghrutam* [one of several medicated ghees given with *snehapana,* made from the five products of a cow].

> Case #2: Reasons for admission: restlessness in mind; childish insistence; angry; sleeplessness; lack of obedience; burning sensation in stomach; extreme thirst. Duration: 2 years.

> Medicines: 1) Special powder—2 × day 2) *avipatti churnna*—alt. days 3) *ashwagandharishtam*—30ml evening 4) *mahachandanadi* oil on the head [prescribed in this patient's case to help with burning sensation in stomach and thirst]. Apply *thailam* if necessary.

The "special powder" is a mixture of equal quantities of powdered *serpagandhi* (a sedative whose Latin botanical name is *Rauwolfia serpentina*), *gokshura churnam* (a diuretic, botanical name: *Tribulus terrestris*), and *swethasanghupushpa* (rejuvenative treatment for the brain, botanical name: *Clitoria ternatta*). Also, according to Dr. Sundaran, ayurvedic physicians use "supporting drugs" (such as *Pipali* [*Piper longum*] and *Haridra* [*Cucurma longa*]) to help with digestion and balance the effects of the principal active drugs.

Although I frequently compare ayurvedic and allopathic medical practices, these two systems of therapy should not be considered radically distinct. An emphasis on the use of pharmacopeia to treat psychopathology is shared by both systems, and ayurveda even seems to have influenced allopathy somewhat in this area. The ayurvedic use of *Rauwolfia serpentina* (an ingredient in the "special powder" mixture described above) for mentally ill patients was adopted by allopathic psychiatry after researchers in India introduced this medicine to the allopathic medical community in 1931 (Sen and Bose 1931). After the alkaloid reserpine was identified as the active ingredient in *Rauwolfia serpentina*, psychiatrist Nathan Kline tested this substance on patients at a New York state psychiatric hospital (Kline 1954), and established it as "the first compound to become available as an effective antipsychotic" in allopathic medicine (Kaplan and Sadock 1995). Both ayurvedic and allopathic healers also emphasize the importance of talk therapy, although many lament that they do not have sufficient time to thoroughly engage in this type of therapy in their busy practices.

Although ayurvedic psychiatrists spend more time talking about medicines and physiological interventions such as *talapodichil* in describing their methods of therapy, many say they consider the counseling they provide to be a crucial element of treatment. Dr. Sundaran asserted that, "With counseling alone, I can manage more than 60 percent of complaints," yet talk therapy or psychotherapy was not often employed in the treatment sessions I observed in allopathy, ayurveda or religious therapies, especially in government-run facilities. When working at clinics and hospitals, allopathic psychiatrists and psychologists see many patients and have little time to spend with each one, and ayurvedic physicians are under similar pressures in such settings. During private consultations, however, patients who can afford it receive a longer session with the therapist. This problem is not limited to India or other low-income settings. Institutional and resource constraints in many sectors of the U.S. health care system limit mental health practitioners from providing the kind of treatment they feel is necessary (Rhodes 1991, Young 1995).

Ayurvedic practitioners engage in a style of psychological counseling that differs from Western-style psychotherapy in some of its premises and procedures. Clinical psychology or Western-style psychotherapy emphasizes exploring past events, and the therapeutic encounter takes the form of a doctor-patient dialogue in which, probably due to a more individualistic orientation, the patient does much or most of the speaking and the therapist avoids giving advice. Western psychotherapy is formalized and institutionalized, and features explicit methods that are taught in training institutes. Ayurvedic psychotherapy is not taught through a formal pedagogy although the *Caraka Samhitā* does provide guidance on how to interact with people who are suffering *unmada*. Ayurvedic healers often tell stories and give moral advice illustrated with examples from their own life experience when counseling patients. In describing his approach, Dr. Sundaran explained:

> I do not generally use basic learning from any book or from my academic experience or philosophy. I'm from a very big family, and I have many experiences with many types of people. I have much experience from my family itself. I have some experience with [people who have] problems of intoxication, the problems of alcoholism et cetera . . . I know some [Western/allopathic, clinical] psychologists, but their approach is, I think, very different from mine because they mostly depend on the classical texts or the texts they are learning. But I mostly depend on my previous experience. I generally do not promote the patients. If a patient's arguments are too much against society, I will claim that your argument is wrong with examples and examples and general stories and general events from general family life or from cinema. From popular cinema also I have used examples.

Dr. Rajendra Varma, an ayurvedic doctor who sees patients with mental problems as part of his general practice at Thaikkattu Mooss' Vaidyarathnam Oushadhasala in central Kerala, describes a similar orientation to talk therapy. He says his methods are "self-developed," and he also uses stories from his personal experience to help his patients develop insights: "sometimes we will tell them, I also had such a problem in my early childhood. I recovered from it because I did this and that, to convince them."

Although ayurvedic psychiatrists listen to the patient and their relatives describe their problems, the doctor spends more time speaking to the patient. In an appraisal of his experience with Dr. Sundaran, a patient I will call Suresh explained:

> Kavitha: Do you talk to the doctor about your problems for a long time? Does he tell you about your problems?
>
> Suresh: Yeah, he talks a lot. I get relief from his talk itself.
>
> Kavitha: You get relief.
>
> Suresh: He talks. His talk is very loving.

Likewise, in Dr. Abdu's consultations at the GAMH, we see a teacher-student style of interaction in which the therapist gives advice to the patient.

Hamid came with his mother and another relative to see Dr. Abdu about his problems, which included trouble sleeping and eating, exhibiting excessive anger, and *manassinu vishamam* (sorrow, mental troubles). After asking about the history of Hamid's illness, his family and social life, and other therapies he had tried—a set of topics that resembled my own inquires with patients—Dr. Abdu gave Hamid some pragmatic advice accompanied by a reminder of his familial responsibilities:

> You have not been able to look after your mom, right? That's a big responsibility, right? You need to support her. That got neglected. That's an important responsibility/great blessing, right? Later, when you get married and all, if you are living in a family, all problems will be solved, right? Then there's the matter of a job. Besides tailoring, you're interested in masonry work, right?

Then, concerned that Hamid is melancholic and spending too much time alone, Dr. Abdu advises him to be more socially engaged:

> Speaking about humans, they are social beings, not meant for sitting alone. We can live only through contact with others. Without that, you know we cannot live. We cannot move a single step without the help of others. Everyone wants people's help. Otherwise, nothing would be possible, would it? If we need a job, if someone doesn't give us one, how will we get one? Nothing will work if one does not get involved with others.

Allopathic psychiatrists and psychologists are normally trained to avoid giving advice in this manner. The aversion to advice and the ideal of equality in the doctor-patient relationship—which one finds in psychiatric texts but less often in practice in India—fits a more individualistic orientation to the self inherent in Western psychological epistemologies. The therapist should assist patients to develop their own insights rather than impart the therapist's views and moral judgments. In India, where the self is not exclusively socially oriented but is more embedded in social ties, it is acceptable to give advice, and it is appropriate that the doctor should act as an authority who can guide, even admonish, the patient. While allopathic psychiatrists and psychologists in Kerala are trained according to a putatively universal approach to the psyche that assumes an individual self, they adjust their practice to the more socially oriented local context and to their own instincts of appropriate social inter-action. For example, one psychiatrist stressed to me the importance of the involvement of the family in therapy in India and explained that he normally tries to enlist a family member as an ally in his treatment of a patient. Likewise, Langford (2002) has shown how an authentic, interior, individual self is elusive in a psychotherapeutic practice she examined in India. The naming of an emotional state, such as anxiety, by the therapist appears as an end in itself, and the therapy focuses on giving advice, "moral caution" or talking about how to deal with social problems related to the distress (246–258).

The more social orientation in India entitles the healer to become involved in the patient's life through giving advice, judging and, if necessary, scolding, but this entitlement also derives from the hierarchical nature of the doctor-patient relationship, which relates to the doctor's professional and educational prestige. In the case of Hamid whom the more senior Dr. Abdu reprimanded for not taking proper care of his mother, age difference is a significant factor in the doctor-patient hierarchy.

In addition to the Government Ayurveda Mental Hospital, Dr. Sundaran's private practice and the Vaidyarathnam Oushadhasala, ayurvedic treatment of psychopathology is also practiced by a few Namboodiri (Brahmin) families of ayurvedic practitioners in Malappuram District, northern Kerala. One of these families resides and practices at their large family estate, Poonkudil Mana, which they converted into a clinic. These *vaidyans*—an often-used classical name for an ayurvedic physician, which is appropriate since these healers are self-consciously "traditional"—learned ayurveda from family apprenticeship rather than through study at a college, and they practice a style of ayurveda that they say is more pure and traditional than that which is practiced at most government and private institutions. Their techniques for healing psychopathology, however, appeared to be quite similar to those employed at the Government Ayurveda Mental Hospital, which is about 20 miles away, although they make their own medicines, and they supplement their medical care with the practice of *mantravādam* ("magic/sorcery"). No other ayurvedic physicians I met claimed they had this capability of using *mantravādam*, and some explicitly condemned this claim as irrational and contrary to what they see as the scientific spirit of ayurveda. Thus, while healers at Poonkudil Mana performed rites to remove malign magical influences, other ayurvedic healers preferred to disabuse patients about their beliefs in possession and *mantravādam. Mantravādam* is normally practiced by esoteric ritual specialists who are available in many communities, and differs from forms of healing that appeal to the divine at temples, mosques and churches.

Allopathic Psychiatry

Along with "English medicine" and "modern medicine," "allopathy" is one of the most commonly used terms in India for the medical system that is also known as "biomedicine," "Western medicine," or "cosmopolitan medicine." "Allopathy" also best characterizes this medical practice in relation to ayurveda and the religious therapies as the term refers to the treatment of illness by opposites, reflecting an approach that involves attacking an illness—for example, using toxic substances that will kill a disease pathogen—and employing invasive techniques. Allopathic medicine is likewise seen as aggressive by many in India. Its treatments are considered powerful and heating, which has positive and negative connotations: allopathic treatments can be highly effective, bringing quick relief for many problems, but the powerful medicines can be dangerous, presenting the possibility of unwanted and injurious side effects. Allopathic medical services, including psychiatric facilities, are broadly accessible in Kerala due to the state's public health programs which have made medical facilities available on even the village level while in many other rural areas of India, people have to travel far to visit a doctor. [15]

For decades now, "Western" medicine has been the cosmopolitan medicine of most regions of the world, and the practice of allopathic psychiatry in India is similar to the practice of this form of healing in other places. Farmer's (1992) analysis of biomedical psychiatry in Haiti reveals an awareness among Haitian psychiatrists of a dissonance between the middle-class, Euro-American assumptions in biomedical psychiatry and the context in which they were practicing. These therapists thus attempted to adapt their practice to the cultural, class and religious backgrounds of their patients—for example, by utilizing explanatory styles from voodoo religion. Farmer claims that this marked ability to discern cultural contingency stems from a Haitian revolutionary tradition of looking skeptically at European ideologies. Allopathic psychiatry likewise has unique traits in Kerala, although psychiatrists there showed less of a critical consciousness of this difference than did their Haitian counterparts.

Western biomedicine arrived in India in the seventeenth century, but was confined to the practices of physicians who worked on ships and in factories for the British East India Company, primarily to maintain the health of company employees. In 1763, after the East India Company expanded across Bengal and other parts of northern and eastern India, the Bengal Medical Service was established, and in the 1860s sanitary commissioners were added to this service to expand public health programs (Arnold 2000: 58). In the early nineteenth century the Company developed training programs that combined European medicine and ayurveda, but this was discontinued in 1835 because of a change in colonial education policy that had begun to assert the superiority of Western knowledge and encourage the explicit promotion of allopathic medicine over ayurveda as a separate and superior science. In southern India, Christian missionary groups, such as the London Missionary Society, played a major role, along with the colonial state, in promoting Western medical

practices. In nineteenth-century Travancore, the colonial-era princely state
that later became part of the state of Kerala, Western medical practices had the
support of the Travancore royal family, whose members used Western medicine and promoted allopathically based public health programs (Nair 2001;
Desai 2005: 468–469). In the early twentieth century, public health programs
in Travancore received further support from the Rockefeller Foundation
(Nair 2001: 222). As in Bengal, promoters of Western medicine in Travancore
encountered local medical practices including ayurveda, siddha and unani,
among which "Ayurveda was the most organized and systematized branch of
medical knowledge" (226).

It is difficult to date the origins of ayurveda in Travancore and the Malabar
Coast, but one study cites evidence of something like ayurveda in this area in
the earliest centuries of the first millenium, while tenth-century inscriptions
indicate the existence of native, hospital-like institutions attached to Hindu
temples (Devi 2006: 73). With the Travancore royal family, missionaries and
the colonial state abetting the ascendancy of Western medicine, ayurveda lost
its dominance as the most established form of medicine sometime around the
late nineteenth century (Nair 2001: 226). In an effort to reinvigorate ayurveda
at the turn of the twentieth century, the Travancore government created a
Department of Ayurveda and founded ayurvedic medical schools (Nair 2001:
227). Thus, from the 1890s to the present, the local governments in Kerala/
Travancore have supported both ayurvedic and allopathic institutions; later
but to a lesser degree, the local governments also endorsed the practitioners
of homeopathy, a medical system that originated in Germany and became
popular in South India. Private ayurvedic schools and pharmaceutical producers, such as the Arya Vaidya Sala corporation, were also involved in efforts to
reinvigorate ayurveda in the early twentieth century (Varier 1996).

The promotion of Western medicine in princely Travancore included treatments for mental illness. Founded in 1870 in Trivandrum, the Peroorkada
Mental Health Centre continues to operate as one of Kerala's largest mental
hospitals, and was one of the primary allopathic research sites in this study. The
practice of clinical psychology in Kerala was initiated in the 1950s by a Keralite,
Dr. V. K. Alexander, who did his training at Princeton University in the United
States and trained the first Ph.D. in clinical psychology in Kerala, awarded
in 1968 to Dr. R. Jagathambika who continues to have a thriving practice
near Cochin in the central part of the state. In the latter half of the twentieth
century, the availability of allopathic medicine was expanded throughout the
state by Kerala's leftist governments, and as described in Chapter 1, people
in Kerala today have greater access to allopathic care than residents of other
Indian states.

Much of the discourse and style of allopathic medicine is shaped by its Western and colonial origins although it has also developed context-specific features as practitioners adapt it to the local setting. Dr. K. A. Kumar, a senior psychiatrist at Trivandrum Medical College who has practiced in Kerala and in the United States, explained that the primary difference he saw in psychiatric practice in these two contexts is that there is a greater involvement of the family in treatment in Kerala. This distinction was cited by other psychiatrists, based on what they had heard or read about psychiatry in the United States, and it struck me too as being the most salient local feature of allopathic psychiatric healing in Kerala. Most patients visited treatment centers accompanied by one or more family members who did much or most of the talking and who are also counseled as part of the treatment. Dr. Kumar explained that he explicitly attempted to determine which family member would serve as the best catalyst in treating a patient's illness. That is, he would identify and work with the person who would be the most appropriate mediator between the ill person and other family members, someone who could also act as a facilitator inspiring the patient to follow his treatment regimen and overcome her problem, which could just as well be a family/community problem.[16]

Family involvement is, of course, a concern in psychotherapy in the United States and elsewhere, but what distinguishes psychiatry in Kerala, at least as compared to the United States and European contexts, is the degree and explicitness of family involvement: one or several family members normally accompany a patient during therapy sessions, therapy decisions are often made by the family, and counseling is often directed at the family group. Nunley (1998) similarly asserted that "[i]n India, then, most information psychiatrists have about their patients comes from members of patients' families," and, as a result of this broad involvement in a patient's therapy, "[t]here is relatively little confidentiality in Indian psychiatry . . . A few psychiatrists provided therapeutic justifications for this lack of privacy, but most of these seemed to me to have the flavor of post-hoc apologies for what is actually a culturally grounded status quo" (329).

In addition to the central role of family involvement in psychiatric therapy, pathological behaviors related to eating mark a difference between the practice of psychiatry in India and normative, Western psychiatric texts and discourses. A psychiatrist at the Trivandrum Medical College pointed out that the *International Classification of Diseases* diagnostic manual, which they use, mentions that anorexia or obesity can be complicating factors in several syndromes but observed that such eating disorders are rarely seen among patients in India. Pathologies related to the consumption of food are present in Kerala, but these included playing with food, taking a long time to eat or delaying eating, and suspecting that foods have been poisoned. I cannot claim to be able to explain this difference in eating behaviors, but I suspect it may be useful to investigate the degree to which they relate to issues of control over oneself as opposed to concerns about the behaviors of others, although surely both orientations are involved in all types of eating disorders.

Some have claimed that a *guru-chela* relationship, a hierarchical relation wherein the knowledgeable and authoritative guru teaches the disciple, exists between therapist and patient in psychotherapeutic practices in India. As mentioned earlier, this style of encounter marks ayurvedic psychiatric consultations, as in the case of Dr. Abdu's consultation with Hamid, and Vaidyanathan has even asserted that this relationship is "the paradigm of *all* relationships in India."[17] Although I observed this style of relationship in ayurvedic therapy, it was less frequent or less explicit in my observations of allopathic psychiatric and clinical psychology consultations. Some older male therapists, however, did occasionally assume this style of relationship, which led me to wonder to what degree the *guru-chela* interaction is implicated in gender relations. I frequently saw older men engage in this teacher-student dynamic in conversation, in therapeutic and other settings, while women of many ages and levels of prestige appeared more interactive in their conversational style.

Allopathic psychiatry is more widely available than ayurvedic psychiatry in Kerala and throughout India, although it is difficult to quantify how much care is provided by general practitioners of ayurveda who occasionally treat mental problems. Most large cities in Kerala have a government-sponsored Medical College that provides psychiatric services. In addition, there are three large, state-run Mental Health Centres, primarily for inpatient care of people suffering serious psychopathology, as well as a number of private psychiatric clinics and hospitals located throughout the state. In terms of health expenditures for the State of Kerala, allopathic medicine receives the greatest amount of government funding followed by ayurveda and then homeopathy (although homeopathy is rarely used for psychiatric problems). Government information on the availability of health services in Kerala, which is reproduced in Table 1, reveals that allopathy has far more beds and doctors but about the same number of facilities as ayurveda in the public and private sectors.

I interviewed patients and healers at three allopathic psychiatric centers: Trivandrum Medical College Hospital, Peroorkada Mental Health Centre and JJ Hospital. Most of the research on allopathic psychiatric therapy was carried out at Trivandrum Medical College Hospital, a large government-run teaching hospital in Trivandrum, south Kerala, which serves several hundred patients in its outpatient facility and has a small, 10-bed female-only inpatient ward. Peroorkada is a large state-run facility on the outskirts of Trivandrum

Table 1.   Health Infrastructure of Kerala.

Medical System	Facilities	Beds	Doctors
Health Infrastructure of Kerala—Public			
Allopathy[18]	1,249	42,438	9,998
Ayurveda	686	2,309	621
Homeopathy	405	950	621
Other Systems	0	0	0
Total	2,340	45,697	11,240
Health Infrastructure of Kerala—Private			
Allopathy	3,565	49,030	6,335
Ayurveda	3,925	1,301	4,130
Homeopathy	421	2,078	2,168
Other Systems	95	139	100
Total	8,006	52,548	12,733

Complied from: State Planning Board *Health Infrastructure and Development Indicators* (1996), in Dr. V. S. Mani "Major Mental Health Issues in Kerala." Paper. Kerala Mental Health Authority (1998).

Note: This data comes from Kerala government sources, and information on some types of healers is not available. For example, the temple, mosque and church discussed in this chapter are not officially considered part of the health infrastructure of Kerala.

that offers outpatient services and wards that can accommodate 500 male and female inpatients. JJ Hospital is a small, private mental hospital in Trivandrum that provides outpatient services and accommodates about 20 inpatients at a time. These hospitals are staffed by psychiatrists and medical students who consult with and treat patients as part of the training for their Diploma in Psychiatric Medicine. A variety of middle-class and poorer patients patronize the Medical College Hospital and Peroorkada Mental Health Centre, where the treatment is free and the cost of medications is subsidized. The private JJ Hospital treats patients from higher socioeconomic backgrounds.

Outpatient care at these facilities consists primarily of consultations with doctors and the administration of medications. During the first consultation with a new patient, the psychiatrist spends 30 to 40 minutes listening to the patient and accompanying relatives or friends describe the characteristics and history of the patient's illness. Like biomedical psychiatrists in North America and ayurvedic psychiatrists in Kerala, they assess the physical health of their patients and perform cognitive functioning and memory tests to account for any physical or neurological disability before making a tentative diagnosis. Psychiatrists use diagnostic categories from the *International Classification of Diseases—10th Edition* or ICD-10, which is similar to the *Diagnostic and*

Statistical Manual (DSM) used by mental health professionals in the United States. The ICD is allegedly an international, culturally-neutral version of the DSM although medical anthropologists have long been skeptical of such claims about the transportability of what they see as Western assumptions about psychopathology to other parts of the world—and we have already seen some cultural discrepancies in the application of biomedical practices in Kerala.[19]

This is not to imply that the ICD is not useful to psychiatrists in India or to deny that there are resemblances in pathological behaviors across cultures. In fact, changing patterns of sleep and relations to food are of keen interest to both ayurvedic and allopathic psychiatrists in assessing the mental health of their patients and in discerning diagnoses such as depression, *vishadam*, and *kaphotmadam*.

After a psychiatrist assigns a tentative ICD diagnosis, he starts the patient on a regimen of medication. Consistent with Nunley's (1996) observation that psychiatrists in India rely heavily on the use of drugs, medication was prescribed for almost every allopathic patient I encountered, and the quantity and strength of medicine given to some patients seemed excessive to some clinical psychologists I spoke with in Kerala. Allopathy is popularly viewed in India as a powerful and heating form of treatment.[20] Allopathic drugs are reputed to have powerful, beneficial effects, but as patients in Kerala show us, this potency can also cause unpleasant and dangerous side effects that have led some patients to seek less abrasive therapeutic alternatives.

The pharmacopeia employed by allopathic psychiatrists in Kerala is the same as that used by psychiatrists in other parts of the world, although the drugs used in India are manufactured by Indian companies under India's Patents Act, which in the case of medications permits the patenting of processes but not the drug products themselves. This has allowed Indian companies to "reverse engineer" drugs and sell them at a fraction of the prices charged by multinational drug companies. However, the process patent provision has been superseded by India's 2005 Patents (Amendment) Act, which was passed to conform to World Trade Organization requirements on patents and may soon prevent Indian companies from manufacturing cheap versions of drugs for which foreign companies hold patents.[21] Fluoxetine, which is produced under the brand name Prozac in the United States, for example, is made by an Indian manufacturer and sold in India under the brand name Fluex at a fraction of what the drug costs in the United States.

The most frequently prescribed psychiatric medicine in Kerala and throughout India, according to psychiatrists I spoke to, is haloperidol, which is normally given to schizophrenic patients, while fluoxetine, which is used for treating depression, is second. Although treatment is free at government facilities, which are widely available in Kerala, and medications are subsidized, poorer patients are sometimes forced to discontinue treatment because they are not able to afford medicines or the cost of travel to treatment facilities. The same is true for patients of ayurveda.

After the initial meeting, consultations with psychiatrists at the facilities I visited are brief, 5- to 10-minute sessions that are largely devoted to medication management. These short sessions are not due to lack of interest on the part of psychiatrists, but are the consequence of a limited number of staff trying to serve a large number of patients. Although patients who can afford to visit psychiatrists in private practice where more time can be devoted to psychotherapy, this should not be taken to imply that private psychiatric treatment is always better: private psychiatry is variable in terms of quality, and the most highly reputed psychiatrists in the state usually work in government hospitals while also maintaining a private practice.

Many allopathic psychiatrists believe that certain patients, such as people they consider chronically schizophrenic, do not generally benefit from psychotherapy and their problems can be managed only through medication. This emphasis on medication over counseling at the government facilities may also relate to the lack of time available for consultation with each patient, and although biological orientations to mental illness are increasingly emphasized in the international community of biomedical practitioners, the emphasis on the use of medication in India is also likely due to advertising, promotion and the sponsorship of research by pharmaceutical companies. Indian pharmaceutical manufacturers send advertisements and promotional literature to psychiatrists' office, and representatives of these companies appear during outpatient consultations to distribute literature and free samples of their products.

On one occasion a pharmaceutical representative offered me drug samples at an outpatient center. Although I explained I was not a psychiatrist and probably should not have them, he placed the samples on the table in front of me before he left. I kept the packaging containing promotional material, and knowing that free samples are passed on to patients, lightening the burden of paying for medications, I gave the pills to a psychiatrist I knew. Although I feel that psychiatrists today in India and the United States rely too much on the use of medications, I realized that through this act I was reinforcing the use of medications for treating psychopathologies. This small example gave me an insight into how through everyday, often well-intentioned practices, the pharmaceutical orientation to mental illness becomes further entrenched despite the skeptical views of many health professionals regarding the emphasis on these therapies. Pills are extraordinarily easy to use, and it is not hard to understand that an overworked psychiatrist might turn to the samples sitting on her desk rather than go to the library and look for research on, say, cognitive behavioral therapy to treat a patient. Even if she did so, she would probably not have the time to apply psychodynamic therapies in her practice.

Individuals diagnosed with serious mental disorders are admitted for inpatient care, which involves medication, counseling and other procedures. Inpatients are given medications in the form of pills or through injections, and electroconvulsive therapy (ECT) is administered to acutely suicidal patients, extremely agitated patients who are not calmed by other means, or patients who have been psychotic for a short duration and are not responding to medications. ECT appears to be utilized in Kerala more often than it is in the United States.[22] Several former patients of allopathic medicine, whom my research assistants and I interviewed while they were using other therapies, reported receiving ECT while being treated at allopathic facilities. As will be seen in Chapter 5, several patients complained about the unpleasant effects of this procedure and the drug injections they were given, and some switched to ayurvedic treatment, which they found to be less abrasive and occasionally even pleasurable to undergo.

Allopathic and ayurvedic psychiatry share some fundamental similarities that become especially apparent when these treatment systems are compared to religious therapies. A key similarity is that both ayurvedic and allopathic psychiatrists work on manipulating the patient physiologically according to their medical system's understandings of biology. Biological manipulation is not completely unknown in religious therapies, and there may be biological effects that derive from patients' engagement in these therapies—for example, a sense of spiritual comfort or inspiration may affect a person's neurochemistry or help relive hypertension. But this is not as explicit or as important as the ill person's relationship to the divine, which is not usually engaged or given much attention in ayurveda and allopathy.

Religious Therapies

The grouping of the healing practices at Beemapalli mosque, Chottanikkara temple, and Vettucaud church into the category "religious therapies" is somewhat, but not completely, problematic. These could also be conceived as three additional therapies, yet their techniques also overlap with the other therapies. Healers at Chottanikkara Hindu temple and Muslim *thangals* (priests/shamans) occasionally administered ayurvedic medications, and the talk therapy employed by the staff at Vettucaud church resembles the practice of clinical psychology. These three therapies did, however, have crucial features in common such as appealing to the divine for relief from suffering and doing so in an environment that was aesthetically engaging, featuring music, smells, tactile and kinesthetic experiences, and visually engaging settings.

I chose to conduct research at Chottanikkara Hindu temple, Beemapalli mosque and Vettucaud church in order to represent the religious diversity of Kerala, where Hindus are in the majority but Christians and Muslims make up almost half of the population. These sites also constitute three of the most well-known and frequently patronized religious healing centers in the state.

Chottanikkara: Abode of Amma-Narayana

Upon arriving at Chottanikkara temple in Ernakulam District, central Kerala, one is enticed with the appeal "Amme Narayana," calling upon the incarnation of God that is present at Chottanikkara. On powerful public address systems and stereos, cassette sellers outside the temple play devotional songs featuring the prominent refrain "Amme Narayana." On checking into the temple guest lodge, one sees "Amme Narayana" on stickers, posters, and painted signs on the walls of the reception office, and one's first night's sleep at the lodge is ended by the loud, predawn, call to worship proclaiming "Amme Narayana" and praising the goddess. In fact, this invocation and its many musical incarnations are so ingrained in me from my time at Chottanikkara that they begin playing in my head involuntarily as I write this paragraph. "Amme Narayana" calls the attention of the divinity, Amma-Narayana, to whom spirit-possessed or mentally afflicted persons at the temple appeal for relief from their suffering. This appeal and the beneficence of Amma-Narayana, along with a special dietary regimen, the experience of undergoing daily *pujas* (worships, ceremonies), the singing of devotional songs, and the opportunity to cathartically act out have helped mentally afflicted people at Chottanikkara overcome their distress.

Chottanikkara temple is an eminent abode of Amma-Narayana, one of the many Hindu incarnations of the divine. "Amma" refers to the female aspect of the deity, and "Narayana" to the male side of the incarnation. "Amma" also means "mother" in Malayalam and is one of the most commonly used terms for "God" in the broad, generic sense among Hindus in Kerala. "Amma" also appears as other female manifestations of the divine in Hindu iconography including Lakshmi, Devi and Kali. It is the female aspect of Amma-Narayana that is most celebrated at Chottanikkara, and worshippers often refer to the deity simply as "Amma" or "Devi."

I am describing Amma-Narayana here as an incarnation of one, absolute deity or divinity rather than as one among a pantheon of gods and goddesses. The divine has many manifestations, and the problem of naming and characterizing the "absolute" is a significant theme in Hinduism. Western Orientalist and Islamic discourses have often construed Hinduism as polytheistic based on the observation that Hindus appeal to a variety of gods with distinct names and identities in their worship at temples and enactment of rituals. A brief conversation with a Hindu who frequents such temples, however, will usually reveal that all these "gods" are seen as manifestations of the one, absolute deity, which cannot be identified by a single name or set of characteristics. Fuller (1992) explained that "all Hindus sometimes and some Hindus always insist that there is in reality only one God, of whom all the distinct gods and goddesses are but forms" (30), and Eck (1998) claimed that asserting the oneness of God while celebrating multiple personalities and forms is a distinguishing feature of the Hindu style of religiosity (24). In the following description, I will attribute several names to the divine to maintain this representational style.

Those who have recounted the story of the origin of Chottanikkara temple take us back to the days when the site of the present temple was a dense forest inhabited by "tribals," a term used in India for the pre-Aryan inhabitants of the subcontinent. One day, a tribal man named Kannappan brought home a cow, intending to slaughter it for food. His daughter, however, refused to allow him to kill the cow, and soon after this protest she, Kannappan's only child, died. After this tragic loss, Kannappan became enlightened and turned his attention to god. After the goddess Devi came to Kannappan in a dream and revealed that the cow was her incarnation, Kannappan transformed his cowshed into a temple.

After Kannappan's death, the temple fell into ruin, and the region was deserted by its inhabitants until one day a *Pulaya* (low caste) woman who was working in the area sharpened her scythe on a stone, which began to bleed. She alerted people from her town who came to see this remarkable sight, and a Brahmin declared that the *chaitanya* (power, consciousness) of the goddess was present—as we will see later, *chaitanya* is a term one woman used to describe what she attained from her healing experience at Chottanikkara. Thus a new shrine was consecrated, and the idol of the goddess in the temple today bears a small incision that is said to be the wound she received from the Pulaya woman's scythe.[23]

The possessed or mentally afflicted at Chottanikkara number around twenty at any time, and according to the temple staff, they come from all over India although the majority are from Kerala. These individuals are described as being

THREE THERAPIES OF SOUTH INDIA   ~: 69

possessed but are also labeled as having a "mental illness" or "mental problems" by their families and by the temple staff. Thus the idioms of possession and mental illness are used simultaneously at the temple. Most of the people suffering mental distress and their families that I spoke with did not see these two idioms as being in conflict or as mutually exclusive, and many of the mentally afflicted at Chottanikkara had previously visited psychiatric facilities for their problems.

Enforcing a restriction that applies at only a few important temples in Kerala, non-Hindus are not permitted inside the main sections of the temple. All the possessed people I met at Chottanikkara were Hindu. Since I am not a Hindu, there were certain things I could not see, but this did not affect my research as dramatically as I thought it might. I simply had to stand on the outside of a four-foot wall or behind a low bar demarcating the temple boundary during ceremonies, which usually put me, along with a few other onlookers, only a few feet away from the rest of the crowd and able to see everything that was occurring. The only place I could not visit was the central shrine, and much of my information about what goes on there comes from the temple priests and my research assistant, Biju. I was allowed to visit the interior of the temple once, however, when I was invited to a wedding that took place there. Temple priests reported that non-Hindus on occasion have come to seek relief from their problems at Chottanikkara. They were supposedly warmly welcomed, as I was, but they were asked to appeal to the goddess from outside the temple wall. Restrictions barring people of other faiths did not exist at any of the mosques or churches that I visited in Kerala.

Although Chottanikkara temple is famous for helping people with psychological or spirit possession problems, it is not solely devoted to this purpose. Regular worshipers and pilgrims visit the temple daily as Chottanikkara is one of the three most sacred temples in Kerala, ranking just below Guruvayoor in northern Kerala and a little above the Sri Padmanabhaswamy Temple in Trivandrum in the South in terms of prestige and auspiciousness. Chottanikkara is also an important site on the southern Indian pilgrimage circuit especially for devotees who are making their way to Sabarimala, a temple in the mountains 90 kilometers from Chottanikkara that receives close to 20 million visitors over the course of its three-month pilgrimage season. Regular patrons and pilgrims are aware that many possessed people frequent this temple, and it is striking to see worshipers nonchalantly carrying out their *pujas* (rituals of devotion) while the possessed are "acting out" around them. While a possessed person is writhing about and yelling on the main temple walkway, other devotees will casually step around or over him. The mentally afflicted are allowed to engage in emotional outbursts and erratic behavior while they also follow a structured schedule of *pujas* and devotional singing.

A distinctive characteristic of large Hindu temples is that, unlike churches or mosques, they are not single structures. A Hindu temple is often a complex of buildings or a campus that can encompass several acres. The main complex at Chottanikkara includes a number of shrines, a dormitory and office building for the temple staff, and a main shrine containing a sanctum sanctorum where the principal idol of Amma-Narayana is located. The main shrine is surrounded by a large, open, gravel-strewn area and a stone walkway that goes around the main shrine. Near the western wall of the main complex stand shrines to Shiva and a snake deity. The western gate of the main complex faces the main road where buses drop visitors from the nearby city of Cochin. The eastern gate of the main complex faces several merchant stands that sell cassettes, books and refreshments and a stone staircase that descends to the temple's water tank where devotees bathe. Further eastward, beyond the tank lies the *kizhakke kavu* (literally, "eastern sacred grove"), which is essentially a smaller temple within the Chottanikkara temple complex and an abode of Kali, a tough, aggressive incarnation of the goddess who intimidates the spirits possessing the afflicted and helps drive them away. (Figure 1 provides a view of the main complex from the eastern gate of Chottanikkara temple.)

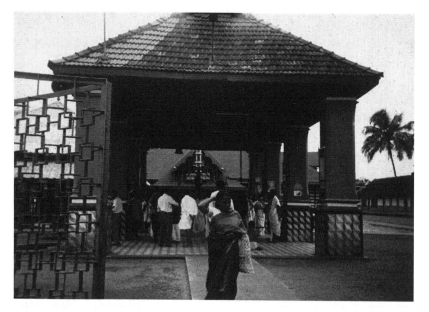

Figure 1. The main shrine at Chottanikkara temple, viewed through the eastern entrance of the main complex. (The people shown here are not among the possessed or ill.)

Each day the possessed and ill supplicants at Chottanikkara engage in an elaborate routine of ritual activities. Most mentally afflicted people reside at the temple lodge, which is where my assistant Biju and I stayed when we were visiting. The afflicted devotees wake up at 3:30 in the morning to convene for a *bhajan*, a devotional song. They then enter the temple when it opens at 4 am, circumambulate the main shrine with the regular worshippers, and visit the other shrines around the temple as they please. In the main shrine, the possessed devotees queue up along with other worshipers to do *darśan*, a mutual encounter with the deity through the image of Amma-Narayana. *Darśan* involves an exchange of gazes between the devotee and the goddess via her personification in her idol in the shrine, and through this encounter supplicants experience the auspiciousness and beneficence of the deity.[24]

Like patients in ayurvedic medical facilities, afflicted supplicants at the temple are required to follow a special dietary regimen. No coffee or tea is consumed by the afflicted devotees in the morning, and around 8 am they are given *ghee* (clarified butter) to drink, sometimes mixed with *brahmi*, an ayurvedic psychiatric medicine, and *panchgavyam*, a mixture containing the five products of a cow that is also used in ayurveda. *Brahmi* is an ayurvedic "brain tonic," made from the plant *Hydrocotyle asiatica* or *Bacopa monnieri* (Dash and Junius 1983: 103). The use of *brahmi*, not just to treat psychopathology but also for the enhancement of mental capacities, has become somewhat fashionable throughout India.[25]

The next event of the day for the patient-devotees, as well as for other visitors, is the 11 am *puja* at the Siva shrine on the western perimeter of the temple. On one of the days I observed the Siva *puja*, I was standing outside the temple, looking over the short temple wall at a small crowd that was gathering around the Siva shrine, a small stone building near the temple wall about 10 feet tall and 20 feet by 10 feet at the base. My research assistant Biju, appropriately shirtless and wearing a *dhoti* cloth with decorative fringe from the waist down, had joined the possessed devotees and other worshippers who were huddled together, eyes fixed on the small door of the shrine waiting for a priest to emerge and begin the *puja*. During this time, possessing spirits became active in three women in the crowd who started swaying gently and then gradually began to dance around. While one of the three women—or the spirit possessing her—began shouting unintelligibly, a man who was also possessed began dancing about, then fell to the ground and proceeded to roll himself around the temple on the temple walkway. Performing an act that some supplicants offer as an expression of extreme devotion, he circumnavigated the main shrine in this way.

While the possessed man made his way around the main shrine, the crowd at the Siva shrine was offering and receiving *prasad*, which consists of food, coins and other offerings that are exchanged between devotees and the deity via the mediation of the priest. The dancing, waiting and exchange of *prasad* had been going on for about 40 minutes when a priest emerged from the shrine on a ledge above the crowd and scattered *dhara* (water, grain and *tulasi*, a sacred and medicinal plant) and flower petals over the devotees. The crowd then slowly dispersed, but gathered again a few minutes later to circumambulate the main shrine as a group. On some days, a few possessed persons would remain, collapsed and motionless or still rolling around on the ground near the Siva shrine after the *puja* had finished.

After circumambulating, devotees leave the temple, and it is closed for a few hours. The mentally afflicted devotees have lunch and then retire to their rooms at the temple lodge for a rest. After the temple reopens at 4 pm they circumambulate the main shrine with other devotees and visit other shrines on their own. An hour or so later, *deeparadhana,* a worship involving waving lights before the icon of Amma-Narayana, takes place in the central shrine, and at 7 pm another Siva *puja* is performed after which devotees join in an elephant-led procession around the temple.

Two nights a week, a ceremony for the possessed and mentally ill is held at the *kizhakke kavu,* the separate, smaller temple to Kali that is just east of the main temple complex. The *kizhakke kavu* is a compound that has no walls: it is sheltered by a roof supported by pillars and is open on all sides. The large, canopied space of the *kavu* contains a small shrine, a space in which the possessed, worshippers and onlookers gather, and a tree that is studded with hundreds of nails. *Kuruthy,* as the evening ceremony at *kizhakka kavu* is known, opens with the beating of drums by temple drummers. As the drumming continues, priests pour water that has been colored with turmeric and lime to look like blood on the base of a small tree that is said to embody Kali. Possessed persons who become engrossed in the drumming allow the spirits to fall into them—the spirits awaken or re-enter their possessees, who then begin to shake their heads, sway or dance about. Some possessees casually hop up and down in place while others cathartically thrash around on the floor. My impression of this performance concurs with Nabokov's description of a similar healing ceremony in the neighboring state of Tamil Nadu as being "like plunging into another, more urgent dimension of human yearning, one in which frantic agitation, passionate enthusiasm, and ecstatic self-absorption are permitted and encouraged" (2000: 78). In the Tamil ritual, drumming was also used to—in Nabokov's terms—"stir" the possessed, underlining the importance of aesthetic engagement in effecting the healing experience in both these settings.

Biju and I had several extended discussions with a 30-year-old man, Rajan, who works at the temple lodge and was once possessed at Chottanikkara.

Rajan spends most of his days in and around the temple and the lodge, and gets to know many of the afflicted devotees. He explained to us that possession begins with a "shock:" "we see someone and suddenly get a fright, it [the spirit] will come inside the body, just like that." He later compared the onset of possession to the experience of "when someone scares us from behind," but "[t]hen what 'depression' [the English term was used] we would feel. That is, that 'depression' is the first thing we will feel." The experience of possession then brings a sense of weightlessness and tiredness after which "[i]t will shake the whole body. Your head will completely thrash about." He added that one loses complete control over the body and consciousness, although one retains some awareness—about ten percent, he specified—of what is going on.

Although Rajan recalled a cathartic possession experience and Nabokov observed "passionate enthusiasm and ecstatic self-absorption" in the Tamil exorcism ritual, it was the female possessees who danced about the most and were more active and demonstrative during possession ceremonies at Chottanikkara. This reinforces studies in various cultural settings that reveal that women more often become possessed or they act out and make their possession more visible.[26] There is no completely satisfying explanation as to why this is so. It is possible that possession constitutes a space of protest or an opportunity to complain about marital, family or social problems in a socially sanctioned idiom. It is true that this is one public realm in Kerala society where women are more active and men more passive, but there are a variety of other ways in which women assert their positions and empower themselves, ranging from the domestic setting to work relations to electoral politics. It may also be that in the ceremony at the *kizhakke kavu*, women feel some affinity with Kali, the fierce, protective, female deity who presides over the ritual and responds to the needs of the afflicted.

In the *kizhakke kavu* ceremony, the participants appeal to a fierce, aggressive incarnation of the divine, known as Kali. Although she is powerful and destructive, she uses her power to protect people from malign forces, and thus the possessed invoke Kali to come down and (wo)manhandle their spirits, to scare them and chase them from their bodies.

My assistant Biju asked Rajan, the lodge worker who was formerly possessed at Chottanikkara, "How does it change [*marunnathu*]?" (using a Malayalam idiom *marunnathu/maruka*, "change," to describe a positive effect of therapy that can imply an improvement or resolution) meaning something like "How does it end?" or "How does the possession episode resolve?" Rajan responded:

It changes "automatically." After a while, we will collapse, we will fall down. [. . .]
We will be really tired, really tired for ten minutes. Then we will become "fresh."

The body will not be weak. The body will get something. Then we will become "fresh." It's difficult to withstand [referring to the experience of possession, the experience of suffering affliction], but after that, we will not know what happened in our body. We will be very "fresh." (Translated from Malayalam, but words in quotes were said in English.)

Rajan's explanation depicts a very sensory, visceral transition from the suffering of possession illness to a freshness in the body that comes with the resolution of the possession experience. But then Rajan explains the importance of the role of the spiritual and religious force (*chaitanya*, the power and benevolence of the deity that supplicants often refer to might be the best term for this), activated by all the *pujas* and ceremonies at the main temple and the *kizhakke kavu*, to transform the affliction:

That itself [doing the *pujas* at the temple and chanting the names of the gods] will make us "pure automatically." Then when the body gets "purified," the "spirit" inside the body will "spread" and come outside "automatically." Then they cannot survive outside. When we pray like this, they cannot withstand it. Then, what happens is, one way or another, they will have to leave.

This is what happens if all goes well following the regular routine of devotion and healing. In some cases where spirits are more intractable, a spirit will demand that a nail be pounded into the tree at the *kizhakke kavu* before they will leave. The spirit will speak through the person it is possessing and specify the length of the nail that should be used. The afflicted person is then taken to the tree and a nail of the specified length is positioned with the patient holding the flat end of the nail to his or her forehead. Thus, symbolically, the nail is pounded into the tree with the forehead, although in practice, the nail is placed with the forehead and then pounded in with a coconut.

Some people I spoke to in Kerala, including some allopathic doctors, reported that they heard of an "inhumane," "barbaric" practice at Chottanikkara where people who are ill are supposedly forced to pound nails into a tree until their foreheads bleed. Similarly, some allopathic and ayurvedic doctors claimed that at Beemapalli mosque the possessed are whipped and flogged to get the spirits to leave their bodies. Some of these things may have occurred, or these may be apocryphal stories used to discredit these places as healing centers. No one who reported these practices had actually visited Chottanikkara or Beemapalli, and I neither saw nor heard any evidence of such beatings or abuses in my observations of practices and interviews with ill people at these sites. Ironically, the only complaints I did hear regarding what one might consider "violent" therapeutic practices related to electroconvulsive therapy (ECT), which is used at allopathic hospitals. Several patients complained of adverse or painful effects of ECT wherein electricity is passed through the body at a level high enough to cause a seizure. Side effects of ECT range from short-term memory loss to broken bones to death from cardiac arrest. No patients I spoke to reported extreme physical injury, but some discontinued allopathic psychiatric therapy because of the unpleasant effects of this treatment.

Dr. Krishna Iyer, an allopathic physician who lives near Chottanikkara and has served on the temple board explained to me that he thinks the temple is an effective place for healing because it engages all the senses: it features a scenic setting, music, fragrances of flowers and incense, and a special diet. I would add that tactile senses are engaged by walking barefoot on sand and stone—while shirtless if one is a male—and having sandalwood paste smeared on one's forehead while possessed devotees who dance about and roll on the ground are kinesthetically engaged in the ritual healing process.

This sensual setting constitutes an important feature of therapy especially for people with intractable problems that have recurred over several years. Although such individuals may never obtain a complete cure, a complete eradication of their illness despite having sought treatment at mental hospitals and other healing centers, they may experience some relief while engaging in healing practices in the aesthetically compelling environment of a religious setting. This amounts to living in the process of therapy as a way of "resolving" a mental problem. Indeed, what one sees in examining the details of the healing practices at Chottanikkara is the sensory stimulation that is engaged. Patients enter the temple at dawn, flowers and water are sprinkled on them, they follow an elephant around the temple, they appeal to Kali and dance about to drums in the evening. And after all this, according to Rajan, the possessee feels very tired but is soon reinvigorated with a sense of "freshness." Although it is hard to appreciate this experience without undergoing this process oneself, we can gain some insight into the nature of this experience by considering how the settings and practices at Chottanikara differ from the relative sensorial sterility of clinic and hospital settings.

There are many other smaller, less well known temples where one can seek relief from possession or psychopathology. Many in Kerala go to local neighborhood temples to pray for relief from a variety of problems, such as a relative who has cancer, a financial crisis, infertility, exam pressure or mental distress. At these temples, people do *pujas* for their problems ranging from a simple and inexpensive flower offering to the elaborate and often expensive *ganapathy homam*, a ritual homage to the elephant-headed deity Ganesh, who is known as "the remover of obstacles." Although Chottanikkara is somewhat distinct featuring a large, elaborated and widely reputed program for people who are possessed or have mental problems, some smaller temples engage in healing practices that resemble those at Chottanikkara.

A small temple in the neighborhood where I lived in Trivandrum held an annual ceremony during which possessed people pounded nails into a tree just as the afflicted do at Chottanikkara. At this temple, the priest also became possessed by the goddess (Amma, Devi)—a fortuitous, auspicious type of possession—and advised people about how to overcome their illnesses or other troubles. Nabokov (2000) investigated the practices of similar healers, known as *cāmis*, in the neighboring state of Tamil Nadu. Just like the neighborhood priest in Trivandrum, the typical Tamil *cāmi* would beat drums, sing praises and use other means to induce "states of trance so as to forecast people's futures and diagnose their sicknesses. Furthermore, he [referring to a particular *cāmi*] could exorcise the evil spirits that had 'caught' them" (19). The *cāmi*, or the goddess speaking via the entranced *cāmi*, would also give personal advice to the afflicted, usually oriented toward convincing the afflicted to conform to the norms of behavior in Tamil society (43). Possession rituals at Chottanikkara, on the other hand, were not so personalized. Rather, afflicted supplicants at Chottanikkara performed *pujas* and possession rituals as a group, though particular possessees and spirits might demand more ritual attention than others. Temple priests did not appear to ever advise individual supplicants about how to transcend their problems, yet other devotees, such as Rajan the formerly possessed lodge assistant, became acquainted with and encouraged the afflicted in their efforts to overcome their problems.

Whether one visits a local temple or undertakes a longer journey to Chottanikkara depends on the severity of the problem and how much time and money one is able to spend. The temple in my neighborhood was patronized by working-class and poor people, many of whom likely would not be able to afford to travel to and pay for lodging at Chottanikkara, which was four hours away by train. There were, however, a few indigent supplicants at Chottanikkara who had found a way there and were sleeping outside near the temple grounds and lodge, and some working class families stayed in the lodge.

Beemapalli Mosque, Where Ummachi is Buried

At Chottanikkara, the mentally afflicted appeal to the goddess in the form of Amma, Devi and Kali while at Beemapalli mosque the ill invoke the name of Ummachi, the female saint who is interred at the mosque. Beemapalli mosque is located in the city of Trivandrum in southern Kerala in a predominantly Muslim neighborhood of the same name. When my assistant Biju or Kavitha and I would visit Beemapalli, we would meet at Trivandrum's bustling East Fort bus stand to begin the half-hour ride out to this coastal neighborhood. Our bus would make its way through the eastern section of the city's old town, which is centered around the grand Padmanabhaswamy Temple, and head out toward the airport. Skirting the edge of the airport, we would occasionally see a plane on the runway, usually a flight heading to or returning from Mumbai or the Persian Gulf, hints of a world of much greater material wealth than the one we were traveling through. We were heading toward the Muslim and Christian neighborhoods that line the coast near Trivdandrum. These neighborhoods are poorer than much of the rest of Trivandrum, yet class differences are not as radical in Kerala as they are in the rest of India. The bus soon came in sight of the Arabian Sea and headed south down the coastal road through the neighborhood of Beemapalli. The trip would come to an end as the bus veered through the entrance of Beemapalli mosque from the coastal road and came to a stop in the large, open sandy grounds of the mosque.

The mosque is an impressive sight after the drive through the modest neighborhood of Beemapalli with its small concrete homes and thatched huts. The building is close to 300 feet in length with 60-foot minarets, surrounded by acres of open, sand-covered grounds where devotees, merchants and numerous stray goats mill about. (Figure 2 shows Beemapalli mosque viewed from the mosque grounds.)

After leaving the bus, Kavitha or Biju, whoever was accompanying me, would head to the mosque's office with me to greet the general secretary, or we would walk through the grounds looking for patient-devotees we had met before or new visitors we could speak to. Along the perimeter of the grounds are lodgings for people who are visiting Beemapalli to find relief from illness, and set off a short distance from the lodgings lies a building with six cells in which violent or agitated possessed or mentally ill people are incarcerated and attended by a close relative. The six cells face an open sandy area at the back of the mosque where, in the shade of a large tree, agitated or violent people are allowed to spend time outdoors under restraint. One person at a time is attached by an ankle chain to a metal post with enough slack in the chain to allow them to walk around in the area under the tree. People with less serious problems—those felt not to be a threat to other ill people or worshippers— wander freely on the mosque grounds. The mosque contains a prayer room for male worshippers most of whom come from the local community to do *namaz*, the Muslim daily prayer cycle. Women and people of other faiths, including some mentally afflicted Hindu supplicants, visit the separate, larger prayer hall, which is oriented around two sarcophagi located behind a glass wall with retractable curtains.

According to Secretary Maheen, the affable director who I would often visit when I arrived to conduct research at Beemapalli, the origin of the mosque centers around the two people who are interred in these sarcophagi: Umma and her son. Ummachi, the honorific but affectionate version of her name everyone uses, was a Mother Teresa-like figure who came to South India hundreds of years ago, allegedly from somewhere in the Levant, to aid the poor and the ill. Ummachi traveled around southern India, and when she passed away she was buried in Trivandrum. A mosque was later built at the site of her grave, a smaller structure that preceded the current building that was erected in 1962. Beemapalli is thus reminiscent of shrines of Sufi saints that people visit for healing in other parts of India and Pakistan.[27]

The majority of people suffering illness at Beemapalli come from nearby districts of Kerala although many visit from the neighboring districts of the state of Tamil Nadu, the state border being only about 15 miles away, and a few devotees make it down from other parts of the country. Most visitors at Beemapalli are Muslims who visit the mosque to pray, but a large number of people of different faiths come seeking help for health problems that range from heart disease to infertility to psychopathology. According to mosque officials and my own estimates, the number of people appealing for relief from illness at Beemapalli at any time is around 150 to 200, of which the possessed and sufferers of mental distress number close to thirty.

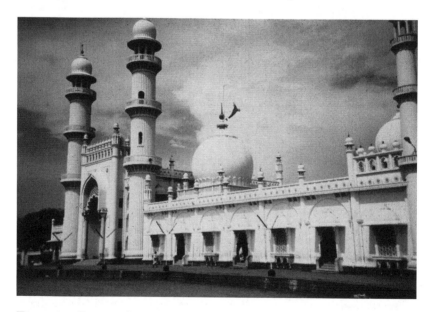

Figure 2. Beemapalli mosque.

Secretary Maheen claimed that a majority of the non-mentally afflicted patients at Beemapalli are Muslim while most mentally ill people at the mosque are Hindu. This kind of syncretism was seen among the patient-devotees who my research assistants and I interviewed at Beemapalli. Eight of the afflicted persons we interviewed were Muslim, seven were Hindu and two were Christian. It was intriguing to hear a Hindu mother who had been living for years at Beemapalli with her possessed daughter explain, while gesturing towards the heavens with the mosque in the background, that her daughter will find relief when Amma—the term for the female incarnation of the divine invoked at Chottanikkara temple—wills it. Our interviews repeatedly affirmed that it was not so much the system of healing or the religious ideology that was important to patients and their family; they were primarily interested in finding a place that would give them some relief and that would do so without causing much discomfort or financial hardship.

Therapy at Beemapalli consists principally of praying, eating jasmine flowers and drinking water from an underground source at the mosque that is said by devotees and mosque officials to have medicinal properties. Other rituals are performed, such as reading incantations and tying talismans around the wrist, but relief is sought chiefly through prayer for assistance from Ummachi and Allah/God. Healing is somewhat more esoteric, the course of ritual and prayer determined largely by the afflicted and their families. In contrast to the organized, group-oriented daily routines of Chottanikkara, ill people at Beemapalli wander the mosque grounds and pray on their own.

My assistants and I asked people suffering mental distress and their attending family members when they thought they would find relief from their problems, and many answered that it is up to God or Ummachi. Some ill people and their families pray and wait for a dream that portends recovery or improvement in their condition. Hanifa is a 30-year-old Muslim manual laborer who had worked in Saudi Arabia for five years and was suffering psychological problems including sleeplessness, "tension" (Hanifa used the English term) and "running off" (disappearing for periods of time without telling anyone). After having been treated at an allopathic mental hospital but finding no change in Hanifa's condition, Hanifa and his wife had been coming to Beemapalli for the last year and a half. Hanifa's wife said her husband's illness has improved since they have been at Beemapalli, and when Kavitha and I asked when they might get relief and leave the mosque, Hanifa's wife explained:

Umma showed us in a dream. [. . .] We will dream about it and in the dream we are given medicines, an "operation" and all. If we dream that we are going home, we can go home. We dreamt of being here until the flag hoisting [a festival at the mosque that was a few months away]. So after that we can go.

In addition to the religious syncretism at Beemapalli, we see here a hint of medical syncretism in the use of the English, biomedical term "operation" in connection with the healing process they are undergoing at the mosque. The wife soon after referred to the jasmine flowers they eat at the mosque as a *kshayam*, a local Sanskritic term for "medicine" also used in ayurvedic discourse. Hanifa's therapeutic regimen also included circumambulating the mosque, bathing in medicinal water from the mosque's well, and oiling his head with a special oil. The oiling of the head recalls the ayurvedic treatment *picchu*, described earlier, in which medicated oil is applied to the head; but there is no indication that ayurvedic medicines were used, and this is not a widespread practice at Beemapalli. This may have been a lay attempt to cool the head or an example of people attempting to apply a pseudo-ayurvedic treatment at the mosque. Recall ayurvedic psychiatrist Dr. Sundaran's observation that some faith healers administered ayurvedic medicines but did not do so correctly.

The most celebrated event of the year at Beemapalli, the Urus festival, is especially significant for people suffering illness. During the week of Urus festivities, thousands visit Beemapalli to pray, socialize, shop at the merchant stalls that are set up for the festival, and attend concerts and other events. At this time, the mentally afflicted and people who are seeking to overcome other adversities circumambulate the mosque carrying one or several *chandanaku-dam* pots (small pots containing incense and coins covered with paper and tied with a string of flowers) on their heads. After circumambulating the mosque several times, supplicants enter the mosque and offer the pot and its contents at Ummachi's tomb. The money in the pots is turned over to the mosque's charitable foundation which, among other projects, is planning to build an allopathic clinic for the neighborhood—demonstrating that the mosque's board does not see appealing to the divine and medical approaches to health as mutually exclusive though there is no indication that mental health facilities will be available at the planned facility.

On the grounds of the mosque, off to the side of the main building is a small structure where people receive prayers and talismans. I rarely saw this facility utilized, however, and none of the ill people or their relatives mentioned visiting this area in describing their healing and worship experiences. On one occasion, I did observe an agitated man who appeared to be possessed standing in front of this small building, muscles tensed and shouting sporadically while a priest prayed over him. Eventually the priest tied a cord around the man's upper arm, which appeared to calm him somewhat. He then walked out into the sandy area of the mosque grounds, and a crowd assembled as he began shouting again, this time more intelligibly, about money and how he feels it controls people's lives.

Although the healing routines at Beemapalli were less structured and programmatic than the routines at Chottanikkara, healing at Beemapalli was a "pleasant," aesthetically engaging process. The outdoor setting at the mosque was visually impressive—a large, scenic structure with spacious grounds, the Beemapalli mosque compound was one of the largest open spaces in the crowded city of Trivandrum. Incense and jasmine flowers brought further sensory stimulus, and although music was not as ubiquitous as it was at Chottanikkara, the plaintive, melodic calls to prayer and the recorded and live music played during festivals provided aural engagements that are not encountered at clinical settings. Vettucaud church, a few miles up the coast and set right on the beach looking out on the Arabian Sea, likewise offers an aesthetically engaging healing environment.

Vettucaud Church

The father of a mentally ill young Hindu man we met at Beemapalli explained that he had intended to take his son to Vettucaud church but after reaching the East Fort bus stand he felt a last minute compulsion to go to Beemapalli instead. This switch is easy to make as the buses to these neighborhoods leave from the same section of the East Fort bus stand. The bus to the Christian neighborhood of Vettucaud also takes a route that is similar to the Beemapalli bus except that after the airport the Vettucaud bus turns right and heads up the coastal road. For this Hindu father, it may have ultimately made little difference which place he chose to visit. He may simply have wished to try the "medicine" of another religion, and, like many families we met, he may be motivated by a pragmatic willingness to give anything a try in the hope that it may help. The term for "mosque" and "church" is, after all, the same in Malayalam. They are both known as "palli." "Beemapalli mosque" is just "Beemapalli" in Malayalam, and Vettucaud church is known as "Vettucaudpalli." These two creeds that came out of the traditions of Abraham look somewhat similar from the point of view of Hinduism, and there was a time when Christians, Jews, and Muslims on the Malabar coast were seen as a single community "of the book" (Ghosh 1992).

The location of these Muslim and Christian communities recalls this past when these religious traditions arrived across the sea that the neighborhoods now face in waves of trade, in the case of Islam, and proselytization, in the case of Christianity. These neighborhoods today maintain a relation to the Arabian Sea as well as to the city of Trivandrum: Beemapalli with its marketplace of imported goods flown over from the Persian Gulf and the Christian communities with their reliance on fishing, which provides the city with its much-loved fried fish and fish curry.

A number of churches and other Christian institutions are located in the neighborhood of Vettucaud and nearby Veli, the most famous being the Catholic Madre de Deus Church. Popularly known simply as "Vettucaud church," this place of worship serves as a refuge where the ill and afflicted seek relief from their problems. As a Catholic church, Vettucaud developed out of a second wave of Christianity that came to Kerala along with European colonialism. Christianity first reached the area in the first century, and these original Christians and their descendants are known as "Syrian Christians" as their faith developed through contact with the Persian church and Syrian immigrants who introduced a Syriac liturgy to the Kerala church. A second wave of Christianity arrived in the sixteenth century with the Portuguese who used coercion and violence to try to convert Syrian Christians to Catholicism. Kerala Christians today adhere to either the Syrian Christian or Catholic faith, and Pentecostalism is growing in popularity in the state.

Dr. V. George Mathew, a University of Kerala psychology professor who comes from a Malayali Christian family and was raised in Trivandrum, recalled for me what he knew of the history of Vettucaud church. He explained that churches in the Vettucaud area were first established by the Portuguese about 200 years ago, and for many years, exorcisms were performed at Vettucaud church, although the Portuguese tried unsuccessfully to stop this practice, which they saw as heretical. Although Dr. George Mathew recalls seeing possessed people at Vettucaud when he was much younger, around 40 to 50 years ago, cases of spirit possession have become increasingly rare at Vettucaud in the last few decades. Today, a number of people with chronic illness problems visit the church or reside in a shed on the church grounds and seek relief from their troubles mainly through prayer or by undergoing counseling with the priest of the church or a nun in the nearby Mystical Rose Convent.

In addition to whatever benefits they may obtain from prayer, people with mental afflictions at Vettucaud, just like those at Beemapalli and Chottanikkara, find some relief or appear better able to live with their problems in the aesthetically engaging environment of the church. Like Beemapalli, Vettucaud church provides a refuge of calm and even a stretch of open space in an otherwise busy and crowded city. As a testament to the spatial and visual environment of places like Beemapalli and Vettucaudpalli, my assistants and I looked forward to visiting the religious healing sites. We found them an enjoyable,

relaxing respite from the busy and stimulating spaces in Trivandrum where we
spent most of our time. Our journey from East Fort culminated in a visceral
feeling of relief and relaxation when we stepped off the bus at Beemapalli and
Vettucaud.

Prayers, the principle means of seeking relief for one's problems at the church,
are performed on one's own as well as at organized services and events. During
the first Friday of every month, hundreds of people arrive at Vettucaud church to
line up for a chance to touch the feet of the statue of Christ outside the church
and visit the shrines inside. Many Hindus join the Christian worshippers who
file past the statue of Christ on First Fridays. All the patient-devotees I met at
Vettucaud were Christian, and I am uncertain whether Muslims ever visit the
church.[28] (Figure 3 depicts Vettucaud church on a First Friday.)

Considering the pastoral counseling offered by the priest and nun at
Vettucaud, it would be fair to say that, at least for the patients who spoke
with Father Hyacinth and Sister Deshiyas, this church placed more emphasis
on talk therapy than any other healing center in this study, and the method
of counseling as it was described to me bore a resemblance to "Western" or

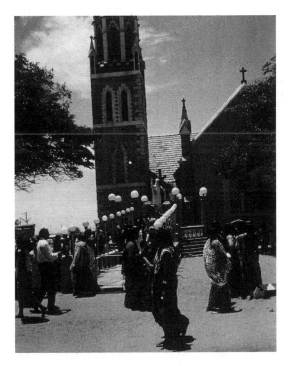

Figure 3.   Vettucaud church during a First Friday worship.

allopathic-style psychotherapy. The counselors at Vettucaud explored the personal, psychological concerns of individuals suffering illness, emphasizing to a significant degree the interior, private realm as the locus of the authentic self.

After relating a Biblical story in which Jesus leads a Samaritan woman to discover her sins, Father Hyacinth, the priest at Vettucaud who provides therapeutic counseling, explained:

> This [Jesus' interaction with the Samaritan woman] is also a therapy: when we begin to talk to the person, we accept whatever they say. If you are going to argue with them, and they know that what they are saying is not correct, you spoil the situation. So rather, when I begin to accept you, you feel that you are happy.

When I told Father Hyacinth that his emphasis on refraining from giving advice and his avoidance of judging the patient reminded me of psychotherapeutic encounters, he concurred but explained that he also intervenes more directly and advises the patient later in his therapy sessions:

> Accept the story, and from the story, guide them where they have gone wrong or where they have been cheated. Place the blame on somebody else, and then bring them to a position where they begin to accept their situation. After that, you can correct them. Before that, if you correct them they will not get corrected.

Father Hyacinth's emphasis on allowing the patient to first develop his own insights calls to mind Kirschner's (1996) assertion that there is a continuity between classical Christian and contemporary psychotherapeutic ways of knowing the self.[29] Although Father Hyacinth explained his willingness to "correct" the patient, ayurvedic therapists appeared more assertive and less equivocal about judging and advising their patients.

Other Therapies

While the institutions and medical practices just described do constitute distinct healing approaches to a certain degree, these centers and systems often have contiguous relations with other healing practices. Meanwhile, people who might be considered mentally ill or distressed pursue relief from their problems at institutions that are not solely or explicitly therapeutic. For example, half a mile from Vettucaud church lies the Divy Shanti Ashram, a charitable institution for the poor that is run by the Vettucaud church organization. Divy Shanti offers food, lodging and prayer services for indigent and ill people and is not an explicitly therapeutic institution. Yet people with a variety of problems including mental difficulties can find a certain kind of relief there having a place to stay and eat while finding solace in prayer and singing sessions. My assistant Kavitha and I interviewed a middle-aged man with psychological and family problems who was staying at Divy Shanti having previously been an inpatient in a mental hospital. He claimed to get some relief from his troubles by staying at Divy Shanti. He was given work to do around the ashram which seems to have helped his self-esteem, and perhaps more significantly, the ashram was a refuge from his abusive siblings.

Also while allopathy, ayurveda and religious therapies are the three most popular treatments for mental suffering, people pursue relief from mental affliction using a variety of other methods, some of which are ancillary or "feeder therapies" for ayurveda, allopathy and religious healing. When assessing potential afflictions of psychopathology or possession, many in Kerala and throughout India visit astrologers. Astrology is not necessarily a therapeutic discipline, but it can help one discover the cause or the meaning of a problem and direct one to an appropriate form of therapy. For example, a person may learn that her difficulties are caused by being born under a bad sign or *dosha* (an astrological condition that is distinct from the concept of *dosa* used in ayurvedic physiology). After learning of the astrological explanation, an ill person will usually seek relief at a hospital, temple or other setting, and astrologers often provide referrals to help the sufferer find an appropriate form of treatment. They may suggest that their client visit the local allopathic clinic or consult a *mantravādan*.

A *mantravādan* is a specialist who performs *mantravādam*, which is usually translated as "sorcery" or "black magic." If a person's problems are believed to be caused by someone having used sorcery against the afflicted person or their family, a *mantravādan's* assistance is usually sought to counteract the effects of sorcery. In Malappuram district in northern Kerala where the Government Ayurveda Mental Hospital is located, Muslim priests known as *thangals* perform many of the roles that *mantravādans* perform in other areas. Also as mentioned earlier in the discussion of ayurvedic therapy, a family of ayurvedic *vaidyans* in Malappuram district supplements their medical treatment with *mantravādam* to heal their clients. All these specialists worked to counteract or remove the effects of sorcery. Just as Nabokov observed in her work with ritual healers in Tamil Nadu where "the 'sorcerer' was always *somebody else*" (2000: 45), I was not aware of anyone who claimed to or was alleged to send sorcery although it was often clear whose jealousy might be the original cause of someone's affliction. The jealousy or resentment of a family often was supposed to have, at least indirectly, instigated the problems of possession and related affliction. The mechanism by which this is happens was always unclear—perhaps it was just too awkward to discuss—but the countermeasures that were necessary were more explicit.

However, few of the patients my assistants and I interviewed who had used *mantravādam* in the past said they found it helpful. On occasion, they experienced some relief after *mantravādam*, but their problem usually returned. Even patients who said their problems were due to sorcery did not report that *mantravādam* provided relief. The brother of a middle-aged Muslim man Kavitha and I spoke with at Beemapalli said his family believes that he is afflicted by a spirit sent by *kshudrum* or black magic/sorcery. The family tried *mantravādam*, but it did not help. The brother complained of all the money he feels they squandered on *mantravādans*, and asserted that they will only pursue relief at Beemapalli. This view of *mantravādam* may be affected by the fact that I did not choose a *mantravādan's* practice as a research site, and thus among those who had used *mantravādam* I only met people who had a disappointing experience and had moved on to another therapy.

A new charismatic Christian retreat in Thrissur District, central Kerala, called Divine Retreat Centre, and popularly known as "Potta," offers another healing option for people with medical and psychological problems. The Divine Retreat Centre is a grandiose facility. The compound is like a small, gated city, with lodging facilities, restaurants, allopathic medical services and a huge amphitheater for prayer sessions and sermons. Employees at Potta explained that each week several thousand people come to pray at the center and many stay for a week or more at the Centre's lodges and medical facilities. One worker at Potta claimed that a third of their patrons are "mental patients" or people with drug and alcohol problems, while others come to seek assistance in coping with a variety of medical conditions or other crises. Relief is sought through collective prayer sessions and listening to sermons either in the amphitheater or via TV monitors located in the medical facilities. Only one afflicted person I interviewed had visited Potta, but at the time of the interview she was seeking relief at Vettucaud church. Potta is mostly frequented by people from central Kerala, although the parents of Mary, a patient I met at the Government Ayurveda Mental Hospital who will be introduced in the next chapter, visited Potta to pray for their daughter.

There are a variety of other temples, mosques and churches that possessed people visit for relief, although they are generally not as large or as well-known as Chottanikkara and Beemapalli. At many small, neighborhood temples, patrons regularly come to appeal for divine assistance with their afflictions, and there are a number of self-appointed healers—often referred to as "faith healers"—who have invented a healing philosophy or claim a divine connection. These healers either work out of their homes, or they found ashrams and develop a small group of followers.

People suffering mental distress on rare occasions visit practitioners of homeopathy and naturopathy. While the terms "homeopathic" and "naturopathic" are used in Western New Age discourse to label ayurveda and other non-Western medical practices, in India these terms actually designate Western medical practices that have been locally adopted. Homeopathy developed in Germany and involves the administration of small doses of medication to cue the body to fight illness. Naturopathy, meanwhile, developed in the nineteenth century in California and was later modified in India with an infusion of Gandhian orientations to nature, diet and health. Naturopathic healers say they are able to resolve mental and physical problems through a proper diet of natural, uncooked foods. Other forms of therapy including south Indian Siddha medicine, which is practiced more widely in the neighboring state of Tamil Nadu, and what are known as "tribal medicines" of the indigenous, supposedly pre-Aryan peoples who reside in the mountains of Kerala, are available although I did not encounter people who had used these therapies.

Finally, I will add to this list of therapeutic options a treatment center that was opened by my research assistant Benny Verghese while I was completing fieldwork on this project. Benny was a graduate student in the psychology program at the University of Calicut in northern Kerala when I met him, and he assisted me with interviews at the Government Ayurveda Mental Hospital. In our meetings and discussions of psychopathology and psychiatric pluralism in Kerala, he spoke of his vision of opening his own treatment center that combined elements of different therapeutic systems. By the end of 1997 he had inaugurated his Thanal Institute for Psychological Services, which combines practices and philosophies from clinical psychology, naturopathy, yoga and Christianity. When I last visited the Thanal Institute in 1999, Benny had several patients and a small staff, and he explained that he had successfully helped several patients who had little success in other therapies. Benny's institute can be seen as a representative of a certain type of healing center found in Kerala, one that is eclectic and *sui generis*, combining elements of diverse healing systems. Many towns and cities in Kerala feature centers like this, often started by a healer with training in a particular field, such as ayurveda or pastoral counseling, who incorporates methods from other therapeutic practices, such as homeopathy or reiki.

This introductory gaze at the diverse therapeutic systems of Kerala provides important context for understanding the experiences of patients who utilize these healing systems. The afflictions of patients, meanwhile, speak to the diversity of life events and social practices that are entangled in the world of health and the healing of mental distress. A variety of desires and stresses shaped by local and translocal influences from Persian Gulf migration to marriage aspirations to trying to get ahead in school help precipitate the problems that led people to these healing centers.

Notes

1. Bhattacharyya (1986), Kakar (1982: 251).
2. The dates of these texts are difficult to establish precisely. G. Jan Meulenbeld (1999) offers entire chapters that identify the dates of the *Caraka Samhitā* and *Suśruta Samhitā*, and cites dozens of studies that place these works in this broad range (105–115, 333–357). The *Caraka Samhitā* was originally composed by Agniveśa, possibly as early as 1000 B.C.E. Later, according to the editors of a recent edition of the text, "it was redacted by Caraka" and hundreds of years after that "supplemented by Drdhabala" (*Caraka Samhitā* 1998: vi). Zimmermann (1987) dates the *Caraka Samhitā* and *Suśruta Samhitā* as being "stabilized in the present form at the beginning of the Christian era" (xiii).
3. For a more thorough introduction to these schools of thought, see Radhakrishnan and Moore's compilation of Indian philosophy (1957).
4. *Nyāya Sutra* Book 1, Ch. 1 in Radhakrishnan and Moore (1957: 359). Parentheses indicate parenthetical comments in the original texts, and brackets, "[ ]," indicate clarifications inserted by Radhakrishnan and Moore.
5. My use of terminology regarding "knowing" and "believing" here and elsewhere responds to Byron Good's observation that medical anthropologists tend to use the term "know" to depict understandings of health they are most familiar with and refer to "beliefs" when describing less familiar medical perspectives (1994: 37–47).
6. See Zimmermann (1987) regarding the role of *dosas* in the natural environment.
7. Dash and Junius (1983: 30).
8. Obeyesekere (1992) demonstrates how physicians consult their understanding of ayurvedic theoretical principles when they create medicines in this manner.
9. Kakar (1982: 244–245). Obeyesekere (1982) and Pfleiderer (1983) offer explanations of the theory of psychopathology in ayurveda that are similar to that of Kakar. Weiss (1986) provides further detail on approaches to psychopathology in ayurvedic texts, and Weiss et al. (1986, 1988) have investigated perceptions of health and illness among psychiatric patients who patronize ayurveda. Nichter (1981) shows how ayurveda is used in negotiating psychosocial distress, wherein patients will, for example, visit an ayurvedic physician complaining of sleeplessness or lack of appetite as a way of getting attention or deflecting blame in interpersonal conflicts.
10. The architecture of the old facility made it so that one ward had to be much smaller than the other, and the hospital directors decided to put the male ward in the larger section. In the new facility, the male and female wards are more equitable in size, and a greater number of women are treated than were before.
11. A researcher at the Ayurveda College Pharmacognosy Research Centre in Trivandrum explained that the cost of ayurvedic medicines is rising because land that is needed to grow plants that are used for ayurvedic medicines is dwindling due to urbanization and industrialization.

12. Satya Pal Gupta in his thesis on psychopathology and ayurveda observed, "Unfortunately, except a few, most of physicians in Indian medicine do not follow the *pañchakarmas* of *samśodhana* [the full name of *panchakarma*]. In some provinces, like Kerala, this therapy is still prevalent and is used in treating the somatic and psychosomatic diseases successfully" (1977: 435).

13. This and most other conversations with healers occurred in English, the language of training in ayurvedic colleges and other professional institutes in India.

14. For further details on the characteristics and physiological effects (as understood by ayurveda and Western-style clinical research) of these medicinal plants see Sivarajan and Balachandran (1994).

15. Panikar and Soman (1984), Nirmala (1997) and Ramachandran (2000: 88–93).

16. See also Roland's (1988) work on individualism, the role of the family and psychotherapy in the United States, India and Japan.

17. Vaidyanathan (1989: 161).

18. The State Planning Board report uses the term "Modern Medicine," but I use "allopathy" for consistency.

19. For example, Obeyesekere (1985) and Kleinman (1988).

20. Nichter and Nordstrom (1989), Nunley (1996).

21. The World Trade Organization requires all member states to guarantee product patents for all products. India's earlier patent law provided an exemption from product patents for food and medications, protecting only the processes for making these products but not the products themselves. This section of the law was modified in 2005 to conform to WTO requirements. Legal struggles have emerged over the implementation of the new law and some drugs are grandfathered and will continue to be produced in India, but in the near future Indian companies will be required to discontinue production of many medications, driving up drug prices for consumers in this part of the world (Halliburton, in press).

22. The rate of use of ECT in the United States was around 3% of psychiatric admissions between 1975 and 1986, although a 1993 study of patients who received a diagnosis of recurrent major depression revealed that 9.4% received ECT (Rudorfer et al. 2003: 1867, citing Olfson et al. 1998). Among the patients I interviewed in Kerala, the rate is around 5 to 10%. It should be noted that the last two decades have seen a resurgence in the use of ECT in the United States, after a decline in popularity in the 1970s (Rudorfer et al. 2003: 1867). Nunley (1998) observed a relatively high rate of use of ECT in Uttar Pradesh in North India, and Shukla (1989) claims that the rate of use of ECT in India is higher than in "the West."

23. Compiled from Vaidyanathan (1988) and conversations with temple priests.

24. See Eck (1998) on the meaning of *darśan* and the particularly visual character of much of Hindu religious practice.

25. For example, Members of Parliament have been taking the drug to increase memory and alertness (Nadkarni, Feb. 16, 1997).

26. See Ong (1987) on factory women in Malaysia, Boddy (1989) on the Hofriyati in Sudan, Skultans (1991) on Maharashtra, India and Pandolfi (1993) on southern Italy. Nabokov (2000: 72–73) explains that in nearby Tamil Nadu, it is new brides who are especially at risk of becoming possessed, and that most possessing spirits she encountered were young men who had taken their lives because of unrequited love or families obstructing their marriage plans.

27. See Pfleiderer (1988) and Ewing (1997).

28. Certain cues in dress and ornamentation make it easy to distinguish Hindus from Christians and Muslims, but it is difficult to discern Muslims from Christians in a crowd without meeting individuals and learning their names.

29. In seeing hints of the "Western" self in this Malayali Christian context, I could not help wondering whether individualism and autonomy might be better characterized by anthropologists as involving a "Judeo-Christian" rather than a "Western" orientation to the self.

3

꧁

LIVES AND PROBLEMS

People in Kerala who visit psychiatrists and other healers for mental problems struggle with a variety of pressures, challenges and expectations. They struggle to find the right marriage partner, they worry about doing well in school in a highly competitive educational environment and many continue to be burdened by the stresses and deprivations they endured when they worked as migrant laborers in the Persian Gulf. These people go from psychiatric hospitals to religious healing centers, and vice versa, seeking help for their problems. They visit healing centers such as Beemapalli mosque, the Government Ayurveda Mental Hospital (GAMH) and the Trivandrum Medical College Hospital, and if they do not find a complete "cure," they often find a way of getting relief—or they discover a more satisfying way of living with their problems.

While I was getting to know the world of health and illness in Kerala, the prospect of presenting information about this world in a way that aligns with the theoretical interests of social science seemed like doing violence to the complex reality of people's lives in Kerala, a sentiment many ethnographers develop during fieldwork. The breadth of issues encountered in working with people who suffer mental problems cannot be conveyed in a single academic study, but with the patient narratives as the axis around which this chapter turns, it is possible to present a broader depiction of Kerala culture and everyday life and the multiple and cross-cutting factors that underlie problems of psychopathology.

In an effort to foreground the lives and health problems of people I spoke with, excerpts from interviews will be presented according to the order in which they originally occurred. I indicate connections to issues in other sections of this study and comment on features of culture and the contingencies of life in Kerala as they arise, but I do not splice together quotations extemporaneously to fit into themes. At the end of this chapter, I present an overview of the themes that arise in relating the stories of these individuals. This synopsis is located at the end of the chapter so as not to orient the reading of this material towards these issues and instead to highlight the narratives of illness and the diversity of issues involved in shaping a psychological affliction.

Two patients from each of the three forms of healing—ayurvedic psychiatry, allopathic psychiatry and religious healing—were selected to represent a variety of features that are socially, politically and medically significant in the local context, such as age, religion, gender, inpatient or outpatient status, socioeconomic situation and other characteristics. In addition, an effort was made to include interviews that were particularly rich in detail, contained a variety of perspectives (such as where patients and multiple family members are interviewed) and featured a follow-up interview. Not all these features could be represented in every case, however. The fact that both ayurvedic patients are female, for example, is not indicative of the nature of ayurveda but rather is an artifact of trying to ensure that Hindus, Muslims, Christians, good informants, working class people and others are included in this section.

When presenting a "patient" or "informant," I am, more accurately, relating the story of the person suffering distress and her friends or family members, who accompany the patient during therapy and who often do most of the speaking. This is the manner in which patients presented themselves to therapists and to my assistants and me for interviews. I was immediately tempted to try to interview patients alone, separately from their caretakers, to get what I assumed to be the authentic experience of the person suffering distress. But such a move would amount to editing out culture. It would, for example, partly obscure the contiguous or socially-dispersed self that is presented by patient and caretaker. Although realms of individual autonomy exist in Kerala and aspects of the individual self may have been submerged by my choice of interview style, I felt that by interviewing patients alone I would be imposing an assumption that a truer self is found in a private setting or at some interior level, an assumption that is problematic in India and may well be problematic in any cultural setting.[1] Nevertheless, in some cases, such as rare instances when individuals visited healers unaccompanied by friends or family, interviews were conducted with the patient alone.

Biju, Kavitha and Benny

My research assistants Biju, Kavitha and Benny ask most of the questions in the following interviews. Although I speak Malayalam, my knowledge of the language cannot compare with that of a native speaker who is fluent in the various vernaculars and attuned to cultural sensibilities of interaction. The presence of my assistants made our interviews richer and made the people we spoke to feel more at ease in a place where foreign researchers are unusual and conspicuous. Equally important to their assistance in interviews, Biju, Kavitha and Benny, all of whom had some training or interest in mental health issues, revealed aspects of culture and everyday life in Kerala and interpreted issues that arose in interviews and in other aspects of our research. Because of their important role in interviews and interactions with patients, Biju, Kavitha and Benny require further introduction.

Biju is an easy-going yet enthusiastic man who lives and works and, it seems, knows everyone in the city of Trivandrum. Biju, during the primary research period for this project in 1997, was in his late twenties and worked as a clerk at an ayurvedic medical institute. He had also been exploring other career options, including graduate studies in psychology, enrolling in the civil service and, after completing work on this project, working as a medical transcriptionist. Biju's personality includes strongly developed, opposite characteristics, which is part of his appeal. He is very down-to-earth and yet philosophical, intellectual and interested in new and exotic experiences. He can seem quiet and even dreamy, as if lost in his own world, yet he is warm and socially engaging. Biju's sociability is evidenced by his many friends and connections. As we moved about Trivandrum, we encountered people he knew in every corner of town, and he made this city of one million feel like a village. He is socially savvy but earnest, and often sought after as a negotiator and mediator. People frequently bring along a friend when they have to negotiate anything, from a business deal to a marriage proposal, just as they do when they visit a therapist, and Biju was often picked for this role.

Biju's empathetic and communicative instincts came out in interviews. Patients we spoke to quickly opened up to him, and sometimes our interviews even seemed therapeutic. A few patients we spoke to became friends with Biju, and at their request he met with some of them alone and informally, not as part of this research project, but because they felt they benefited from talking to him.

Kavitha is equally easy-going although not as outgoing as Biju. Having recently finished her Masters thesis in psychology on stress suffered by wives of Malayali men who work in the Persian Gulf, which will be discussed later in this chapter, Kavitha was beginning work on her M.Phil. in psychology while she assisted me in my research. At first, she struck me as a polite, earnest listener who did not offer much information about herself, but this deference at the outset of our relationship was undoubtedly partly related to gender expectations. Women are often expected to be initially deferential in conversation with men, especially in a work relationship, which is not to say that everyone follows this model. I gradually got to know Kavitha well and felt very rewarded by the experience. Behind her quiet, genial manner is a tough, strongly motivated woman who stands up for her convictions. As very few graduate students in India take on jobs during their studies, I was impressed that Kavitha took up the opportunity to work with me when she heard through a psychologist I know that I was looking for an assistant.

Kavitha also had a reassuring and empathetic manner in interviews with people who were suffering distress. Patients we spoke with appeared at ease and often opened up to her. She knew exactly how and how long to listen and when and what to ask—although I also, probably less tactfully, interjected questions and suggested which way the interview should go in many of our discussions with patients. Ultimately, I think people we spoke with sensed that she was sincere in wanting to know their story, and, as with Biju, they appeared to find talking to Kavitha to be therapeutic. I suspect that some patients at psychiatric facilities found our interviews therapeutic simply because psychiatrists were always quite busy and were unable to spend much time talking with patients, while we were able to converse with them for an extended period, listening to the history of their troubles and frustrations.

As I was leaving Kerala in early 1998, Kavitha was beginning her M.Phil. research on suicide, a topic she developed interest in while we were doing our interviews. This is a compelling topic as Kerala has the highest suicide rate in India, and Kavitha is one of the few researchers, in addition to myself (Halliburton 1998), to examine this topic in detail.

Since finishing her M.Phil., Kavitha has worked as a therapist at a drug and alcohol deaddiction and family counseling center and at other institutions. While many psychology graduates in Kerala decide to pursue more lucrative positions outside their field of specialization, Kavitha remains committed to a career as a counselor and a healer.

I met Benny when he was a graduate student in psychology at the University of Calicut in northern Kerala and a part-time counselor at an allopathic hospital near the university. Benny assisted me in interviewing patients at the Government Ayurveda Mental Hospital in Kottakkal. Like Biju and Kavitha, Benny was sympathetic and engaging in interviews, but he was more outgoing and assertive and proceeded at a quicker pace. He had a personality that would flourish in the United States. Energetic and confident, he showed the signs of someone who would become the leader of an organization or at least his own boss. Sure enough, while I was conducting fieldwork, Benny put his studies on hold and opened his own healing center that combined aspects of Western psychology, ayurveda, yoga, naturopathy and Christian teachings.

Benny was a little more insistent, but gently so, in getting people to talk about their problems. Witness the quicker pace and shorter exchanges in Benny's interview with Mary that follows, compared to the exchanges in the interviews involving Biju and Kavitha. Overall, Benny seemed to lead the interview, while Biju and Kavitha would get the patient to lead.

When I left Kerala at the beginning of 1998, Benny had nearly completed building his clinic, which he called Thanal Institute for Psychological Services. On returning in 1999, I found that Thanal, which is in central Kerala in the town of Kaladi, was doing brisk business for a place its size and that Benny was quite busy. Along with his psychologist-assistant and nurses, Benny had a combined caseload of about ten patients at a time. He reported to me that he had success in healing people and was able to help patients who had unsuccessfully sought treatment at other, more prestigious and established clinics.

All my assistants had some training in Western-style psychology, and I wondered to what degree this might influence the course of our interviews and the way we interpreted informants' problems. All three assistants appeared open-minded toward the perspectives of other healing systems, and, in fact, they were all referred to me by friends and contacts whom I got to know because of their interest in diverse forms of healing. Still, there was a tendency in our early interviews to employ allopathic psychological and psychiatric rubrics, to look for "depressive" or "schizophrenic" "symptoms" in our encounters with patients, for example. When I explicitly told my assistants that we should try our best to avoid privileging allopathic and psychological categories and assumptions in our work, I thought they made a good effort to ease up on their psychological perspectives and check their use of psychiatric terminology. Of course, our perspectives surely continued to be shaped by these and other influences in ways we were not aware, but I feel we were able to de-center our western/allopathic psychological assumptions to some degree. My assistants' efforts at open-mindedness at times even led them to "overcompensate" in their perspectives. Each assistant to varying degrees looked critically and skeptically at allopathic psychiatry, and sometimes they celebrated, perhaps romanticized, other forms of healing. Biju, for example, became an enthusiast for the healing rituals at Chottanikkara and was often asking if we could squeeze in just one more trip to the temple. Like Farmer's (1992) observation that Haitians are easily able to see the cultural and class assumptions behind biomedical psychiatry due to the history of class struggle in Haiti, I wondered to what degree Biju, Kavitha and Benny were "natural anthropologists," having grown up in a society with diverse forms of healing, aware of multiple perspectives about illness, perhaps realizing that each is constructed and has its own contingencies.

Sreedevi and Her Mother: The Melancholic Daughter Who Wants to Marry

A 22-year-old woman I call Sreedevi was accompanied by her mother when Biju and I first interviewed her in the office of the ayurvedic psychiatrist they were consulting. Sreedevi's problems included stomach pains, episodes of *bahalam* (agitation or tumult), loss of energy and a decline in interest in her studies.

We interviewed Sreedevi and her mother using prepared, semi-structured interview questions, which focus on the history of the illness and therapy-seeking, reactions to different therapies, opinions about the cause of illness and future plans to get relief from the illness, and we asked additional questions that came to mind as the interview progressed. In our first interview, in January 1997, Sreedevi was quiet, lethargic and unemotional, and her mother spoke for her almost the entire time. In her initial attempt to describe Sreedevi's problems, her mother explained:

> She is not eating, and she has started crying. And when sleeping, she'll suddenly wake up complaining of stomach pain. She shows *bahalam* [agitation/tumult]. There is a doctor near our home. We took her to see her. That doctor had done "psychiatry training." So the doctor said this is a problem. She prescribed some pills and all for my daughter. That's how it first began. It was a year ago. I did it that way because the doctor said to.

> Biju: Is this problem your biggest worry, or do you have any other illness?

> Mother: What's most bothersome now is she'll cry now and then. There is *dukham* [grief/sadness], and this studious girl is no longer interested in schoolwork.[2]

In addition to her sadness and stomach pain, Sreedevi's mother mentions here her daughter's *bahalam*, which refers to agitated behavior or outbursts—for example, shouting and striking things, or "throwing a fit." Sreedevi has also lost interest in her studies. She had finished her Secondary School Leaving Certificate (SSLC), which one achieves after the tenth year of schooling, and she began working on her Pre-Degree Certificate (PDC—a prerequisite to enter a university) in commerce, but as her illness developed she discontinued her studies.[3] At the time of our interview, she was training to be certified as a typist, a less prestigious educational accomplishment than what she had been striving for earlier. Sreedevi's mother is a school teacher, which may explain why Sreedevi went as far as she did with her education and why her mother is distressed about her loss of interest in studies. But such accomplishments and concerns about education are not unusual in Kerala where 90 percent of the population is literate and the state has the highest average number of years of schooling per capita in India.[4] Young men and women are under great pressure to excel in school, and they push themselves—or are pushed by their families—to outdo their peers by hiring tutors or attending supplementary educational "coaching" classes.

We inquired further about the development of Sreedevi's problem, which began with what may have been a somatic expression of distress in the form of stomach pain:

Sreedevi's Mother: For the first treatment, we consulted a doctor for stomach pain. That doctor is a specialist in this area, so she gave this medicine. Then after seeing her [Sreedevi] continue like this, we started consulting another doctor. That doctor referred us to a psychiatrist, a senior psychiatrist. We went to his house at Medical College [referring to a neighborhood of the city near the allopathic Medical College], though he's not connected to Medical College. He gave treatment right in his home. She was taking a pill called Hexidol.[5] It was going on like this [she was just carrying on with treatment and things were uneventful] until finally she asked the doctor, "Will I be able to get married?" So the doctor said, "Yes, you can marry," and he said, "You should inform the husband's family when you get married."

Biju: Now are you using a different treatment?

Mother: Afterwards, she had the problem again.

Biju: Why did you change treatments? Why did you change to ayurveda?

Mother: Well, it was a few days ago that we "discontinued." After that, again . . . Then finally we didn't see the doctor for several days. Then we used ayurveda. Ayurveda is a good treatment. Treatment is like this in ayurveda, but as for the other one [allopathy], there are some "side effects." Because this is a mental problem [*manassikamāyittulla vishamam*], we have been coming here.

Biju: Who told you about ayurvedic treatment?

Mother: I read about this treatment in the paper and brought her here.

Biju: Are you doing the previous and current treatments at the same time?

Mother: No. But they are still giving a pill called "Hexidol."

Biju: Did you have the same symptoms during the previous treatment?

Mother: Yes.

Biju: The previous doctor and the current doctor. Do you agree with the way they understood the illness?

Mother: The two are about the same. I feel they were the "same." Do the two doctors have the same view? Is that what you mean?

Biju: That's it.

Contrary to studies of "hierarchy of resort," or what therapies people use in different contexts, which have found that patients resort to allopathy later in the course of therapy-seeking, an overwhelming majority of my informants in Kerala first sought relief from allopathy.[6] This pattern of therapy seeking may relate to the fact that allopathic care is widely available in Kerala, and its virtues are promoted through the media.[7]

The allopathic doctor Sreedevi originally consulted for stomach pain referred her to an allopathic psychiatrist, who prescribed medication. The problem continued despite this treatment, and Sreedevi and her mother sought assistance from an ayurvedic therapist. This is a common scenario. Most people I met at non-allopathic treatment centers had previously tried allopathy and switched treatments when their problem returned. Those who changed therapies did not do so only out of concern that their condition had not sufficiently improved. Like many Malayalis who choose ayurvedic treatment, Sreedevi's mother says she prefers ayurveda partly because she believes that it has fewer side effects than allopathic treatment.

In the preceding excerpt, Sreedevi's mother identifies her daughter's problem as explicitly mental (*manassikamāyittulla*), which runs counter to current research that claims to have found non-Western peoples expressing distress primarily through the body. People in Kerala demonstrate a concern for states of mind and consciousness that is informed by a phenomenological orientation that values the more intangible aspects of the person. Examining discourses of consciousness, body and self in terms of a local phenomenological orientation yields a more nuanced and complete depiction of the variations of human experience than hoping to find in the nonwestern subject an embodied alternative to the prioritizing of the mind in Western phenomenology.

At the time of this interview, Sreedevi was continuing to take an allopathic medicine called Hexidol while undergoing ayurvedic treatment. Hexidol is a combination of haloperidol and benzhexol hydrochloride, which is normally given to people allopathic psychiatrists consider schizophrenic. We did not investigate Sreedevi's allopathic medical history in detail, but Biju and I were surprised that she was given this drug as she seemed primarily quiet and depressed, more neurotic than psychotic, or in ayurvedic terms, more *kaphotmadic* than *pittotmadic*. Sreedevi's ayurvedic therapist was planning to take her off this drug, but he was doing so gradually.

In response to our question as to whether Sreedevi and her mother agree with how current and previous healers understand her problem, Sreedevi's mother explained that they feel that both the allopathic and the ayurvedic doctors had the same view. Similarly, other informants told us that they agreed with the points of view of all previous healers. It was rarely perspective, belief in a system or conviction about what constituted a "correct" understanding of illness that determined choice of therapy. It was thus more likely the promise of a safer treatment, one that has fewer side effects as she claims, rather than a particular belief in ayurveda that led Sreedevi and her mother to switch to ayurvedic therapy.

With Kerala's highly literate population, many ill people and their families learn about various therapies by reading the numerous articles and advice columns on medical issues that appear in newspapers and magazines. Likewise, Sreedevi's mother says she learned about ayurvedic psychiatric treatment after reading about it in a newspaper.

Sreedevi's mother then considered the possibility that her daughter's problems may have been affected by a failed attempt to arrange a marriage with a young man from their neighborhood whom Sreedevi liked. From her description, it is unclear whether it was Sreedevi's mother (her father is deceased) or the boy's family that did not agree with the marriage proposal. Getting married or finding the right marriage partner, which involves developing relations between families as much as between the individuals getting married, is a major preoccupation among families in Kerala as well as throughout India. It is a constant subject of conversation and the topic of innumerable Malayalam and Hindi films. According to her mother, failed marriage arrangements related to the onset—but were not the only cause—of Sreedevi's problems:

Biju: Do you think the main reason behind this problem is "marriage?"

Mother: Speaking about "marriage," it's not particularly about "marriage." It is from that that this problem developed. At that time we didn't want anything. We didn't make any agreement and all. Between them [Sreedevi and the potential husband] there were no other *bandhanngal* [relations—that is, there was no dating or affair going on].

Biju: What else will you do to get over this illness?

Mother: Like I said, I think her mind must be changed/improved [*mātti*].

Biju: Will you do any other treatment? You've done allopathy and ayurveda. Anything else?

Mother: Particularly, before, the head ... in the "pipe" ... she got a strong blockage. So I wondered if there was some problem with her nerves. I still wonder that.

Biju: Are you thinking of taking her to a "neurologist"?

Mother: Yes. I have thought of doing that. That is to say, because of that, I feel I might do that. I've thought of that.

Biju: Do you have any other plan to get over this illness?

Mother: No specific plan. When this illness started, we took her to a temple, and as is our custom, we took her to a swami who said prayers and tied a string. That was for mental contentment, at Attukal [a temple].

Biju: Are you still going to the temple?

Mother: No. The priest said, go to the Devi temple, and on the second day do *raktapushpārchana* [a ritual offering of flowers]. On the fourth day, do *navagrahārchana* [nine planets worship]. Do all that, he said. For *raktapushpārchana*, there is a Devi temple near us. We have been going there and doing this every Tuesday. Do this 21 times, he said. We have done seven or eight. So we are doing all that.

Biju: How much more time do you have remaining?

Mother: Let's see. A month, a year. We still have four or five months to go.

Biju: What is the next step you will take?

Mother: I want to get over this. I would like my daughter to get married.

Sreedevi's mother explained that they originally went to a temple to see what they could do about Sreedevi's troubles, and a priest recommended they perform twenty-one *raktapushpārchana*, which is a ritual that involves offering a certain kind of flower known as *raktapushpa*. *Raktapushpa* literally means "red flower" and the term is used to refer to a variety of species that produces red flowers.[8] Many people suffering illness perform similar rituals at local temples while also seeking relief through medical therapies. These rituals are not as explicitly oriented toward healing as the ceremonies at Chottanikkara temple though they may have been tailored to Sreedevi's problems and her concerns about marriage. *Raktapushpa* is a red flower, and redness is associated with fertility and, thereby, marriageability in South India. Thus the flower offering may make Sreedevi's marriage prospects more auspicious while helping her psychologically to prepare to find a suitable partner.

The "pipe" Sreedevi's mother alludes to is most likely a reference to *dhumapana*, a therapy the ayurvedic psychiatrist used on Sreedevi. This treatment involves rolling ayurvedic medicines into a cigar, which the patient smokes by inhaling through one nostril and exhaling through the mouth. The ayurvedic therapist explained that this helped to get rid of Sreedevi's hallucinations, a characteristic of Sreedevi's troubles that we did not learn about through our interviews and which may have led the allopathic doctor she saw earlier to prescribe the antipsychotic Hexidol.

Sreedevi's mother says that some way or another Sreedevi's "head"— her mental problems—must be "changed" (*mātti*). "Change" (*māruka*) is a Malayalam idiom that describes what one achieves through healing. "Cure" has no precise translation in Malayalam, and patients speak of their experiences in healing primarily in terms of "change" and "improvement," which imply a more incremental and open-ended approach to healing compared to the ideal of curing. As we will see in Chapter 5, curing aims at complete eradication and a return to normalcy or a pre-morbid "baseline," while "change" denotes the more incremental, partial improvements that are more often the result of therapy. "Change" can also refer to what some patients report as a positive transformation to a state that is more enhanced that one's normal, pre-illness state.

Biju and I conducted a follow-up interview with Sreedevi and her mother in August 1997, seven months after our original meeting. While informally chatting soon after we met Sreedevi and her mother, Biju and I could quickly tell that Sreedevi was doing much better. Her expression was brighter—her flat, melancholic look had faded. She was focused, and she appeared to have more energy. She occasionally spoke and showed interest in the conversation between her mother, Biju and me, but Sreedevi still was not outgoing. We got the impression that her quietness, her shyness, is part of her normal demeanor, but she no longer appeared tired and laconic. Since our last interview, Sreedevi and her mother had been to the Government Ayurveda Mental Hospital in northern Kerala, and Sreedevi underwent the 45-day course of treatment there. They both felt that this experience had greatly improved Sreedevi's condition. The only problem Sreedevi now had, according to her mother, was that she felt she had recovered but was bothered that healers thought she should continue to take medicine in order to fully complete the course of treatment. Her mother explained:

> She has good "change" and all, but she says, "I have no illness at all. Why am I continuing the medicine? Now I have no problem at all." Now when I give medicine, this is the reply. She spoke very little earlier. Now she is speaking very well, going everywhere. She is doing all her work a little "better." That is, after taking the treatment.

> Biju: Have you experienced any improvement or decline in your present state?

> Mother: It is improved.

> Biju: Since we last spoke, what treatment have you been doing?

> Mother: Just this, ayurvedic treatment.

> Mother: [part of Sreedevi's mother's response is obscured by conversation between Murphy and Biju] . . . Kottakkal. Even compared to here, there were differences/improvements [*vyatyāsam*] in Kottakkal.

While earlier Sreedevi's mother used the term *mātti* ("changed"), here she talks of *vyatyāsam*, which means "difference" but can also be translated as "improvement" in the context of healing, and uses the English word "change" to describe what was accomplished in treating her daughter.[9] We then asked Sreedevi's mother to describe the therapy at the GAMH:

> We stayed 50 days there. They gave ghee after cleansing the bowels. Ghee was given for seven days. First, two ounces. Each day, they added an ounce, step by step. It took one week for that, and 14 ounces were given finally. She did not eat anything during that time. She did not take any food. Speaking of that, she vomited. It was coming out from her mouth right while she was drinking. Then after that, after drinking ghee, then after *marupatthyam* [the period of rest and simple diet between treatments], they did *vasti, tailam, kshāyavasti* [enemas and medicines]. That for one week. After the first three days, then *nasyam*. After

nasyam, this was done on the head, like this. They put medicine and wrapped [referring either to the *talapodichil* "mudpack" treatment or the *picchu* oiling of the head described in the previous chapter], and gave two types of medicine mixed with yogurt at night.

The purgative Sreedevi was given is one of the procedures that rids the body of impurities (or "toxins" may be an appropriate biomedical translation) at the beginning of the course of treatment known as *panchakarma*. Sreedevi was also required to drink ghee in amounts that increase by one ounce every day in order to lubricate the body for *panchakarma* therapy. The *vasti* Sreedevi's mother refers to is an enema, and *nasyam* is medicine that is administered through the nose. Both of these are part of the *panchakarma* treatment. The wrapping therapy Sreedevi's mother refers to is *talapodichil* or *picchu*, or it may be a reference to both. In these treatments, medicated mud in the case of *talapodichil* or oil in the case of *picchu* is applied to the top of the head, which is wrapped with a banana leaf or cloth to hold the medicine in place. Several of these procedures are reported by patients of ayurveda to provide aesthetically pleasant, "cooling" effects. Biju then moved on to a question that was included in order to discern whether patients became aware of different symptoms after changing therapies. This did not provide any insights into the suggestive power of different therapies to cause patients to attend to different symptoms as I had hoped it might, but it did get people to elaborate on whether there were any changes in the patient's illness:

Biju: Are there any new symptoms since we last spoke?

Mother: Nothing new. Still, when talking, suddenly words, a blockage . . . they don't come out naturally.

Biju: Do you have any new ideas about your problem? Do you have any sort of new ideas about your problem? Do you have any idea about the reason it began? Anything in particular?

Mother: I don't have anything in particular. I had scolded her a little for not studying. She didn't study in a good manner. She hasn't studied well. She will sleep lying face down. I have scolded her when she shows laziness and all. I don't know whether that made her "feel."

As to whether there were any new ideas about the origin of Sreedevi's troubles, her mother wonders whether she scolded her too much about her studies, again raising concerns about educational success. Also, Sreedevi's mother uses the English term "feel," meaning in this case something like "upset." Two other informants we will meet later, Mary and Hanifa, describe their problems using the English word "tension." A variety of English terms for emotional states have been adopted into Malayalam, both diversifying people's repertoires for expressing distress while possibly displacing some Malayalam idioms. While I am not able to determine whether the proliferation of English language emotional idioms involves a decrease in the use of Malayalam terms for distress, the increase in English emotional terms appears to coincide with a decrease in the incidence of spirit possession as well as a homogenization of the identities of possessing spirits (Halliburton 2005).

Biju asked Sreedevi's mother what problems remained, and what, if any, further treatment needs to be done:

> She is saying "Why is medicine being given to me." That's her opinion: "I don't have anything, doctor." When we saw the doctor here, we were asked to continue for one year, right? That period is about over, right? "Now why should I continue for one more year" she says. She wants to have a family. That's why she wants to know whether it will take much longer. That's one of her problems. "I have recovered due to the conversation. I understood."

Sreedevi's mother repeats that the only problem now is that Sreedevi feels she is fine and is questioning why she has to continue taking medicine. Sreedevi spoke up on this issue herself and told us, "I have been taking medicine for several days now, and I don't know what my illness is." Officially completing her treatment, and the "clean bill of health" that can be claimed from doing so, can enhance Sreedevi's marriage prospects. Families negotiating a marriage often feel compelled to reveal such illnesses and to point out that therapy was completed in order to reassure the prospective family—even though such mental difficulties often reoccur. It is, of course, tempting to hide information about mental illness, but if someone is marrying within their community, which is usually the case, prospective families are likely to learn of such problems through their social networks. Thus it is important to head off such concerns with an assertion that the problem has been treated, and this is what the first psychiatrist was suggesting when he said, as Sreedevi's mother recounted, "You should inform the husband's family when you get married."

The assertion that Sreedevi has recovered through "conversation" is somewhat unique. In most of our interviews with patients of allopathic and ayurvedic therapies, there was little discussion of the counseling that is given—narratives about therapy experiences focus more on medications and treatment procedures such as electroconvulsive therapy or the ayurvedic medicated mudpacks and enemas. This could be because Sreedevi's current ayurvedic psychiatrist has more time to counsel patients. In fact, this therapist told me that he considers the advice he gave Sreedevi and her mother to be a key factor in her recovery. He was concerned that Sreedevi had been idle for five years, not doing any work at home. "I tactfully advised her mother to give her more duties," he recalled, explaining that her mother responded by assigning Sreedevi more responsibilities.

The treatment Sreedevi underwent appeared to be helping. The fact that Sreedevi's desire to get married is making her impatient to finish treatment is, I believe, cause to be optimistic about her future. But more importantly, the mood and manner Biju and I observed on our follow-up interview showed us that, as they say in Kerala, something had "changed" in Sreedevi for the better.

Mary and Her Mother: The Woman Who Wanted to Be a Nun

Mary is a 29-year-old Christian woman who was seeking treatment, accompanied by her mother, at the Government Ayurveda Mental Hospital (GAMH). When my assistant Benny and I met her, Mary was on her fourth visit to the GAMH in three years, this time for attempting suicide by jumping into a well. Her suicide attempt was a response to difficulties that appeared to start when her parents refused to allow her to become a nun.

Early in our interview, Mary explained "I got mental 'tension'" (*Enikku manassinu* tension *vannu*—literally, "mental tension came to me")—invoking an English-language term that has emerged in Kerala to designate emotional distress. Mary did not go into further detail about how she experienced this "tension," and Mary's mother intervened to describe the problem as she saw it:

Mother: One day when she was sad [*vishamam*], she came home laughing.

Benny: She came home laughing.

Mother: Yes. Then one day she came home from work weeping. Then we asked, "Why are you sad, daughter? Why did you come home crying?" She did not answer. Then after that day when she would come home from work, she would act strangely and show *bahalam* [agitation/tumult/throwing a fit]. Then we took her to the hospital.

Benny: When she was laughing like that, did she hit [things or people] and use bad language?

Mother: She swore and said that I was immoral and beat me.

Benny: She will do all that. Is she this way with her father too?

Mother: Yes. Ask her father.

Benny: She doesn't fear anyone?

Mother: No fear at all. When she is angry, nobody knows what she will do. Sometimes she will grab a knife.

Benny: Did she cut anyone?

Mother: No. She never cut anyone. When she is angry, we act according to the situation. She will throw at us whatever she can get her hands on. She will break the door. Then her anger will disappear and she will become calm.

This *bahalam* (outbursts of anger or fits) and use of bad language were frequently reported symptoms among patients we interviewed. (Sreedevi was also described by her mother as exhibiting *bahalam*.) During this admission to the GAMH, Mary was given the diagnosis *vishadam* which resembles the diagnosis *kaphotmadam*. *Kaphotmadam* is characterized by a phlegmatic, depressive and sad disposition, but lacks the occasional outbursts of anger that characterize *vishadam*.

Mary and her mother agree that Mary's problems are to some degree related to her parents preventing her from becoming a nun:

Mother: One reason is that she wanted to become a nun, but we did not support this.

Benny: Who wanted to become a nun?

Mother: She did.

Benny: Mary really wanted this, but it was not allowed.

Mother: So I said, "Daughter, you are my only daughter. Don't go off and do that. That is my opinion." I don't know whether it might have caused her some pain.

Benny: (to Mary) Did you feel terrible when your father and mother told you could not become a nun?

Mary: Yes.

Benny: Do you think that this was the reason for your illness?

Mary: Yes.

Benny: Do you think that because of that God gave you this illness? That God called on you and you did not go.

Mary: Yes.

Mary later had additional complaints about her family:

Benny: What is your problem, Mary? Consider me as a doctor. I am working in a hospital in Kozhikode. My home is in Arulakam [place names are pseudonyms]. My sister is married to [someone in] Mangalapuram. I am telling you this just so you know who I am. Mary, what is your problem? Something is worrying you though you are not showing it on the outside.

Mary: Nothing is worrying me.

Benny: Nothing is worrying you.

Mary: If I get *ati* [hit/slapped/spanked], I am sad.

Benny: From whom? Who will hit you, Mary?

Mary: My father, mother and brothers.

Benny: That may be because you did something.

Benny tries to get Mary to confide in him by revealing who he is. He tells her where he is from and identifies the town his sister married into (her husband is from the town and she now lives there with him) which reveals that Benny is also from a Christian family. Revealing one's home town and one's community ties that develop through marriage are key parts of identifying oneself, and are usually the first topic of conversation when people in Kerala are getting to know one another. After urging her to talk about her problems, Mary reveals her concern about being "hit." The word Mary uses–*ati*–is hard to translate and is worthy of some attention since the way it translates has a variety of implications and raises delicate issues. *Ati* can mean "hit," "spank," "slap" or "beat," and the precise meaning depends on context. In this case, *ati* refers to something like "spanking," a way of disciplining children, but in many cases in Kerala this is done when sons and daughters are older. "Slap" or "hit" is more appropriate since *ati* is often a single swat or cuff on the head. Mary may have actually been beaten or may be traumatized by this hitting/spanking, but that is hard to discern from this statement. Benny interprets that the incident involved a socially acceptable use of physical discipline. Mary then explains that she was scolded while she was praying and that her family hits her when she refuses to eat:

Mary: [. . .] When I am eating, they will hit me.

Benny: Who? Your family?

Mary: My father.

Benny: That will be because you were probably doing some mischief while you were eating.

Mary: I can't eat.

Benny: Do you sit without eating? Then they will hit [*ati*] you. That is because they love you. They don't want you to become too thin. So why are you worrying?

Mother: She's not willing to eat anything.

Benny: Is she reluctant to eat now also?

Mother: Yes. Now also I . . .

Mary: I am eating.

Mother: When I take a stick she will eat.

Refusing to eat is a common symptom of distress and psychological suffering in Kerala, and is taken very seriously. Ultimately, the issue of "hitting" is difficult to engage. I hope that this attempt to translate these incidents does not make it sound like these are barbaric, exotic acts. At the same time, I do not think it is right to over-relativize the situation and assume that what occurs is not painful for Mary or more serious than what is being revealed. We will hear a concern about a form of violence that is unambiguously condemned in Kerala when Mary later reveals that she does not wish to get married for fear that her husband may beat her.

Mary and her mother go on to recount the efforts they have made to find a solution to Mary's problems, which first emerged ten years earlier. For seven years, Mary received treatment from two allopathic doctors as well as from a church "father" who was qualified as an allopathic psychiatrist and treated

Mary with hypnosis.[10] For the past three years, however, Mary has come to the GAMH in Kottakkal whenever her problems return. We asked Mary what specifically led her to seek treatment at the GAMH on this occasion:

> Benny: Now is the fourth time. What is the problem for which you have come here now?
>
> Mary: I jumped into the well.
>
> Mother: She will jump into the well. She doesn't take her pills, and then she takes several pills together. She took four pills at a time. She wants to die.
>
> Benny: Will she say that she wants to die?
>
> Mother: Yes.
>
> Benny: Mary, do you want to die? Then how can you get married? [Mary had earlier expressed a desire to get married.]
>
> Mary: I want to get married, but when I get married, if my husband beats me, I won't be able to bear it.

We did not ultimately learn of the cause of Mary's concerns about domestic violence. She may have witnessed it or experienced it at home, or she may know someone in a physically abusive marital relationship. It is also possible that this is symptomatic of or an aspect of a larger, more generalized sense of distress. On several occasions, Mary shifted the focus of her concerns and undermined some of her earlier claims. Mary's mother then explained that Mary had previously attempted suicide by overdosing on pills. Unfortunately, suicides and suicide attempts are not uncommon in Kerala. The state's suicide rate is the highest of any Indian state and is three times the national average.[11] Mary may be attempting suicide because she feels trapped. Marriage would be a way to get some autonomy from her family members, who scold her, hit her and did not let her become a nun, but fear of being beaten makes her dread getting married.

After learning that Mary had attempted suicide on two other occasions when she was seeing an allopathic psychiatrist, we asked Mary and her mother to explain why they changed to ayurvedic treatment after pursuing allopathic therapy for seven years.

> Benny: So why did you change from allopathy to ayurveda?
>
> Mother: We believe that they can relieve her illness.

Benny: To get relief. Is there any change after coming here?

Mother: There is a great decrease [*kuravu*] in her anger and her attacks on others.

Benny: There is change. Will she do housework since she started coming here?

Mother: She will do the work.

They did not elaborate on what specifically they thought would be different about ayurveda, but like many patients we interviewed who were using non-allopathic therapies, Mary and her mother switched after several years and two or three courses of allopathic treatment. Although Mary attempted suicide again since switching to ayurvedic therapy, Mary's mother believes that Mary is less angry and has fewer violent outbursts. There is no resolution to Mary's problem, but there is "change," as Benny affirms.

Mary and her mother also visited a church in central Kerala to seek relief for Mary's problem. They did not offer details about the healing process, but Mary recalled "when I was treated there, I got *sukham* [health]." She then asserted, "I don't have any problem now" and "I always have peace," which was hard to take seriously given her recent suicide attempt, but these statements about going to church for relief were the most enthusiastic and positive comments Mary made during our interview. Mary also spoke with some frustration about not being allowed to become a nun, and her first complaint about her family was that they scolded her while she was praying. She probably felt some satisfaction after seeking treatment at the church since she had a chance to engage her spirituality. Likewise, being left home while her parents visited a Christian retreat did not seem to help her.

Mary's parents visited a popular Christian charismatic center called "Potta," described in the previous chapter, to seek relief on Mary's behalf, but Mary did not accompany them:

Mother: . . . When we went there [to Potta], the nuns told us that it is not necessary for the patient to pray. Only the father and mother have to pray.

Benny: I see.

Mother: They said, come to this place with a right mind.

Benny: So if the mother and father come to pray that is enough. They said not to bring her to Potta?

Mother: They said not to bring the person who was ill.

Benny: They told you not to bring her. So you, her father and mother, prayed for her.

Mother: They told us not to bring her.

Benny: Then also there is no change [that is, even after praying at Potta, there is no improvement in Mary's condition]?

Mother: None.

We also asked whether Mary and her mother had consulted astrologers or done any *pujas* (offerings at a Hindu temple). Mary's mother explained that they had not because, "Her [church] father said we will never do such things" and because "[w]e have faith" indicating that, although some Malayali Christians use Hindu rituals, they will only engage in Christian worship for Mary's troubles. Affirming her family as an exception to the religious eclecticism and pragmatism we found at religious healing centers, Mary's mother proclaimed "even if she does not recover from her illness, I am not going to do things like that."

Shortly after this assertion—and perhaps motivated by the dissonance between her mother's profession of devotion to her faith and her parents' opposition to her joining the church—Mary began to claim she was adopted:

Mary: These are not my real mother and father. You all adopted me. You did not deliver me ... [followed by something unintelligible].

Benny: What is she saying?

Mother: She thinks that she is adopted by us.

Benny: She is adopted.

Mother: We are not her family. We adopted her. That is in her mind.

Benny: Mary, why did you say this?

Mary: No reason. It's nothing.

Benny: Why? Are they not giving you real love or is it because they did not allow you to become a nun. So then? (Pause.) Why did you say what you said? (Pause.) Mary?

Mother: She will tell me I'm not her mother. She will tell me to go away, and she will say that I am not her mother.

Benny: Do you want me to ask your mother to leave so that I can ask you some personal questions?

Mary: There's nothing. I don't have anything to say.

On a few other occasions during this interview, Mary brought up a complaint or accusation and then retracted it. This reveals a pragmatic feature of this interview. What seemed significant was that these were moments when Mary asserted herself most. For example, she grabbed her mother's and our attention and controlled the conversation in the preceding encounter. This momentary assertion of power may, like her *bahalam* outbursts, be an attempt to feel she has some control, some voice within this family that did not let her follow her calling. However, the fact that Mary at times made assertions only to retract them makes one wonder how performative or manipulative some of her earlier accusations might have been. Ultimately, Mary was hard to read. Sometimes her manner was dramatic and attention-seeking, but she also appeared genuinely distressed. She alternated between appearing to be a victim and a manipulator.

Like all the ayurvedic patients we interviewed, Mary was discharged at the end of the 45-day treatment period. Mary and her mother did not respond to our follow-up inquiry, which we sent by mail. We did not see Mary or her mother again, nor did we hear that she was readmitted to the GAMH. Benny and I hope that no news is good news.

Abdul-Rahman: Homesick in the Gulf, Unhappy at Home

Abdul-Rahman is a 29-year-old, Muslim man who was seeking allopathic psychiatric treatment as an outpatient at the Trivandrum Medical College accompanied by his brother and sister. Biju and I interviewed Abdul-Rahman alone at the Medical College psychiatric outpatient center, and afterward we had an informal conversation alone with his brother and sister. Abdul-Rahman, who like Sreedevi had studied up to his Secondary School Leaving Certificate, was employed in Kerala as a newspaper distributor and also spent time working in Mumbai and the Persian Gulf. Abdul-Rahman returned from the Gulf because he felt homesick, but after returning he became restless, had trouble sleeping and felt *vishamam* (sadness/depression). Abdul-Rahman tried allopathic psychiatry, homeopathy and a Japanese healing system called "Okiyama" to cope with his problems.

Three months before we met Abdul-Rahman, he consulted a psychiatrist near his home town in southern Kerala. Having heard that the doctors are better and the treatment free at Trivandrum Medical College, Abdul-Rahman set out for Trivandrum along with his brother and sister.

When we asked Abdul-Rahman how his problems started, he told us how eight years ago he left Kerala to work in Mumbai, but he found the experience lonely and depressing. "Everyone's life was alone" and "Only friends were there," he recalled, lamenting that he and others he met there were living away from their families and adding that he returned to Kerala because he was homesick.

Biju asked Abdul-Rahman to describe his problems more explicitly, to depict the emotions and experiences he had undergone, and Abdul-Rahman elaborated on the pain of being away from home when he worked in the Persian Gulf. The language in the excerpts that follow is occasionally awkward. This is partly because of the difficulty of rendering Malayalam in English and preserving its style and meaning, but also because Abdul-Rahman had an elaborate and unusual way of speaking. Also, like other Gulf migrants, Abdul-Rahman's English is very good, and his speech was heavily seasoned with English terms:

Biju: What was your illness like? Were you depressed/sad [*vishamam*]?

Abdul-Rahman: I was sad [*vishamam*], a sorrow in the mind. So, I wanted to see everyone, to see everyone from home. It was as if I was alone. Then, after that, I went to Bombay again. After that, I got a chance to go to the Gulf. So I went to the Gulf. I went as a "fabricator," as a "steel fabricator." When I got there, I didn't get even a chance as a welder. As I had some difficulties in the company, I was forced into a bad relation with the "parties" [his employers or the middlemen who got him the job]. I remained with them only one year. After that, for one year I was with my elder brother. So, when I departed I was with my elder brother. Thus mentally, when I remained like that for a long time ... I was getting letters and things from home. Still there were economic difficulties so I remained there in the hope of solving economic problems. Then one day I felt mental sorrow [*manassikamāyittu vishamam tōnni*]. I was crying and could not eat. At that time, I felt that I should simply cry like this, that tears should come to my eyes. When lying down, I would see nightmares. I woke up startled, and then could not get back to sleep. When I became restless/worried [*veprālamāyittu*], I got a ticket to come home and an "emergency passport" and came home to my native place [*nātu*].

After being home for a few days, I had no illness. Suddenly there was no problem. Soon after seeing everyone at home, I was able to eat and everything. My illness was completely changed. After that, now one year later, I again got my old papers from the agency and resumed my old routine. I did lots of work and became very "active." I had the ability and self-confidence to undertake anything. Still now, even when I took the papers from the agency and went to distribute them in the morning at 5 am, after that, while I was doing this, I started a shop, hoping to "progress" and to start a book stall in front of the shop and an agency office. I borrowed money for the shop.

Abdul-Rahman's homesickness is understandable given that in southern India one's "native place," or *nātu* (sometimes transliterated *nadu*), plays an important role in the construction of personhood. Attachment to place is, of course, not unique to South India, but the Malayalam language and people's everyday discourses of identity feature explicit and pronounced articulations of relations to place. *Nātu* has no clear equivalent in English and is usually translated as "native place," referring to the town or region one is originally "from," usually a birthplace or a place that one primarily identifies with as having contributed to one's essence—or "substance-code" to use Marriott's (1976) term that attempts to transcend what he sees as Western dichotomies of form/substance and actor/action. This place attachment is not only sentimental, but can also be visceral, physical and "biological" in the sense that it relates to South Indian views of the body, material substances and the relations between these. Daniel (1984), in a work that is influenced by Marriott's non-dualistic view of the self and "substance-code," claims that people in the state of Tamil Nadu (the name of the state contains the word *nātu/nadu*), which borders Kerala, have a visceral attachment to their native town or land. They feel that the substance that makes up their selves, their bodies and their character also exists in the land of their native place, in, for example, the soil and the food it produces. I heard similar sentiments from people in Kerala. In fact, Abdul-Rahman speaks of home in connection to food. He explained regarding his return to Kerala after working in Bombay, "As soon as I reached home ... right away I had food and saw everyone." Ayurvedic medicine and lay medical knowledge assert that the qualities in the soil of a place are also present in the food and in the bodies of people from that place. When people in Kerala meet, they quickly inquire about the other's "place" (*nātu* or *sthalam*), and they often use place names to further identify themselves in the way North Indians and North Americans use last names or family names. Srivastava (2005), however, argues that in South Asian studies claims of attachment to place are overstressed to the exclusion of discourses of itinerary and mobility, which are also central in Indian cultures. The meaning of *nātu* and the ayurvedic theories of soil and substance should not necessarily be seen, therefore, as indicating an immutable sense of attachment or as exclusive discourses about relations to place. Many Malayalis move away from Kerala for a long period, or permanently, and do not experience the same reaction to displacement that Abdul-Rahman describes.

Regardless of the degree of one's attachment to place, the life of the Gulf worker is challenging. In the past two decades, many have come from India to work in the Persian Gulf countries. Migrants from India usually head to the wealthy city-states of the United Arab Emirates, such as Dubai and Abu Dhabi, or to Saudi Arabia, Kuwait or Bahrain, where they are able to earn far more than they can at home. Although figures are inconsistent, Kerala has the highest rate of Gulf migration of any Indian state, and a sizable portion of Kerala's economy comes from remittances from Gulf workers.[12] While many have reaped financial rewards from working in the Gulf, Indian workers are often exploited. They have to pay usurious fees to middlemen who help them get employment and work permits, and as Abdul-Rahman learned, they do not always get the work they are promised. Additionally, migrants are sometimes not paid for their work, and they have little recourse for fighting such injustices. Still, many successful migrants return to Kerala with significant savings, which they use to raise their level of prestige in the community and to marry into a more successful family (Osella and Osella 2000a, 2000b). It must have weighed on Abdul-Rahman that he did not return from the Gulf a financial success as he had certainly seen other young men do and as has been depicted in Malayali films.[13]

On returning to Kerala from the Gulf, Abdul-Rahman's problems subsided, but after going back to his old job of delivering newspapers and trying to open a shop, his *vishamam* (sadness/depression) returned:

> To tell you the reason I am coming here now [to see an allopathic psychiatrist], later when I was working in the paper agency, there was a weight like this in the mind. I was crying, complete *vishamam* in the mind. Just like when I was in the Gulf, I will cry.

Abdul-Rahman then explained he was upset that he did not get the job he expected in the Gulf, and his employers there were not paying his and other workers' salaries. So they organized a strike "like we do in our place," he said, referring to Kerala's tradition of assertive labor organizing. Kerala's labor unions have significant power, and strikes frequently occur throughout the state. Kerala workers are well paid compared to other Indian laborers, and Kerala's Communist government has generally been supportive of workers' movements. However, Kerala workers' demands for living wages have led industries to move to other states in search of more exploitable labor, and the state now has a high rate of unemployment, which fuels the out-migration of workers to the Gulf and elsewhere.

After discussing his return from the Gulf, Biju and I asked if Abdul-Rahman had tried other types of therapy. He said that during the previous week he took a homeopathic medication, but he did not continue with that therapy because, he said, "it doesn't become suddenly 'active.' I was told to decrease the 'dose' when I take it." Abdul-Rahman's eagerness to get fast results from therapy may explain why he was presently seeking allopathic treatment, and his comments foreshadow a theme that we will see repeated in later chapters. While many in Kerala prefer a treatment that is more "pleasant" to undergo, such as the application of the ayurvedic *talapodichil* "mudpacks," many choose allopathic therapy, along with its side-effects and more abrasive procedures, because they heard it gives quick results. Many are pressured to return to work or school or they feel hurried for other reasons, and the speed of allopathy accommodates these pressures.

Abdul-Rahman told us he continues to use a Japanese healing system called Okiyama, which he started before seeking allopathic psychiatric therapy:

> Yes, it's a treatment system. It's called "divine light Okiyama." It comes from Japan. Divine light. "Divine light." It is a divine light that we cannot see. They give "divine light" . . . That is, they give it to the forehead at first and to the "medulla oblongata." After that they will do it to our important points.

> Biju: Where is this light coming from?

> Abdul-Rahman: We can't see where the light is coming from. The reason is that since my problem must change by whatever means, the first "time" there was some change. Before going to Okiyama, I had terrible restlessness. Before going to Okiyama, I had terrible restlessness and rolling [sic]. So the first day I went to Okiyama for the "first treatment," they gave me "divine light." Having given that the first day, I felt giddiness and swinging in my head. We know that there is only one side to them. They give "divine light" only to the forehead. Thus my head swung and rolled and all that. I fell down. There is a center at Punalur.

> Biju: Isn't God [*daivam*] involved?

> Abdul-Rahman: Yes, God [*daivam*] . . . faith in God [*iśvara*]. They also believe in only one god.

Although some therapies used by people suffering distress, such as ayurveda and siddha, developed in the subcontinent and have been practiced in southern India for centuries, people in Kerala also patronize local practitioners of therapies from other parts of the world, such as homeopathy (from Germany), Okiyama and reiki (from Japan), and naturopathy (from the United States). I did not come across any other description of Okiyama in the course of my research. According to Abdul-Rahman, this therapy bears some similarity to the transnational Japanese healing system known as "reiki," a healing system that is considered "spiritual" and involves the manipulation of energy channels.

At the end of this segment, Biju inquires about the role of God/the divine in Okiyama, using the word *daivam*, and Abdul-Rahman responds referring to the divinity as *daivam* and *iśvara*, both of which are often used as non-denominational terms for "God" in India. However, these terms, being Sanskritic, are also associated with Hinduism. This mixing of religious terms recalls the Hindus suffering illness at Beemapalli mosque who referred to the divine as "Allah" and "Amma," invoking both Islamic and South Indian Hindu names for "God." Abdul-Rahman's sampling of homeopathy and Okiyama and the Hindus who visit Beemapalli testify to the pragmatism in people's therapy-seeking habits. People in Kerala shop around for their therapeutic options, and while some such as Mary's family will only engage with secular therapies (such as ayurveda and allopathy) and religious healers of their own faith, many cross conventional religious boundaries in search of relief from their afflictions.

After Abdul-Rahman described his Okiyama treatment, Biju asked him to elaborate on his illness experience:

Biju: When your illness is intense, what is your problem? Do you get angry?

Abdul-Rahman: Not angry, nothing. When I say I have illness, people at home will say . . . I will say, I don't have an illness. But people at home are terribly "worried" about me. Since I do everything at home, they cannot bear it if I get some problem. I cannot tolerate those sorrows. Usually when I get *vishamam*, I am very restless. Sometimes I will want to lie down, and then when lying on the bed, I will feel the urge to get up . . . no, not to lie down, but to sit down. I want to sit down. When thinking about sitting down, I decide no, I want to walk. When walking, I change my mind and want to come and sit again. When lying on the "left side" normally one turns and lies on the "right side." But when I am lying on my "left side," I will get up and lie on my "right side."

These themes of indecision, restlessness and *vishamam* recur throughout our discussion with Abdul-Rahman. He later explained that when he thought he should sleep, he would be unable to and would just continue turning over in bed.

We then asked Abdul-Rahman to further explain his experience with allopathy and Okiyama. When asked about his allopathic treatment, Abdul-Rahman launched into a narrative oriented around medication, naming the different pills he took and the different dosages he was given at different times:

Biju: How do you "feel" when you are taking "allopathic medicine"?

Abdul-Rahman: Speaking about allopathy, it's either "tablet" or "medicine." If it is the other one [probably referring to Okiyama], there is nothing to just take inside or apply on the outside of the body. At that time, if I was taking pills . . . When I first took Trika, I completely recovered. I "stopped" it myself. I stopped. Later, it was December 30, at that time, the doctor scolded me a lot and prescribed a more powerful drug. He prescribed Amitriptin C+. I "continued" that. Then I was prescribed Anxit 5 mg. After that, my illness decreased for several days. Then, again, it increased. It increased again, and when I went to see the doctor he prescribed Trika for me. For the Trika, he first prescribed 1 mg. The illness decreased for several days. When it decreased, later on I went to see the doctor who gave me 5 mg. He gave me 5 mg. When again it decreased, I didn't go to see the doctor. In the meantime, later on, one day, it was my "sister" who went to see the doctor. I got the illness again that day. When my "sister" went to see the doctor, I took a pill. Since Trika was not available, I had Anixit 5. Now when I take Trika, there is a restlessness in my body. At that time, I had more of a problem. I was in such a state, I couldn't bear the dosage. But it was not possible to take it at home.

Patients of allopathic medicine commonly offered medication-oriented narratives like this in describing their treatment. Medication is usually emphasized over psychotherapy in Kerala due to the biological orientation of contemporary allopathic psychiatry, the marketing and promotions of Indian pharmaceutical companies, and the fact that doctors have little time to meet with patients at government health centers. Here Abdul-Rahman says he was given Amitriptan C+ (amitriptyline) which is used for insomnia, anorexia and depression, Trika (alprazolam) which is prescribed for anxiety and panic attacks, and Anixit 5 (another brand of alprazolam). In our discussion with Abdul-Rahman's brother and sister, his sister listed the same medications, and confirmed that these medicines helped at first though their effects wore off over time. This excerpt ends with a comment on adverse effects Abdul-Rahman experienced from allopathic medications—Trika caused restlessness and effects he "couldn't bear" at a higher dosage he was taking earlier. Such concerns about unpleasant or abrasive effects of treatments were almost exclusively related to allopathic medications and procedures. Recall Sreedevi's mother's concerns about "side effects" in allopathic therapy in explaining her preferences for ayurvedic treatment.

In contrast to the medication-oriented recounting of his allopathic therapy, Abdul-Rahman's description of Okiyama is more embodied and experiential—this might seem to be the result of Biju asking him to describe the therapy in terms of his "feelings," using this English term, but Biju asked about allopathy using the same terms:

Biju: What were your "feelings" when you were taking the Japanese medicine?

Abdul-Rahman: Now there are no "feelings" for that. The first time I had "Japanese treatment," when I went there and they gave the "divine light," my "body" totally turned around. I fell down. Even though I collapsed, I was conscious. I have a memory of everything I did, but I could not control my body. I turned around and around and fell down. Though I had fallen down, they kept giving "divine light." When they gave me this, I fell down. It was like this the first time. The second time it was less. The third time . . .

Biju: How did this affect you?

Abdul-Rahman: After this there was no problem. Though they were giving the "light," they gave it with my body sitting like this. Now there is no problem, no problem for my body.

We then inquired whether Abdul-Rahman would consider trying any other forms of treatment in the future:

Abdul-Rahman: Whatever may be the treatment, I only wish to recover completely.

Biju: What treatment are you most interested in trying? For example, going to ayurveda, a temple or a mosque?

Abdul-Rahman: Well, generally, I don't have any preference. Whatever may be the form, I only want to get better.

When we asked whether he preferred allopathy or Okiyama, Abdul-Rahman gave a similar answer: "By whatever means, I want to get better [*māri*, lit. "change"]." This is another affirmation of the pragmatism and flexibility about using different systems of medicine that was highlighted earlier. People we spoke with did not appear to wrestle with the issue of which therapy was "right," which belief system they should agree with. In response to questions about future plans for therapy, we often got answers like those Abdul-Rahman provided: that is, the ill person and family were willing to try whatever might work. This flexibility is consistent with observations made by other researchers who found that therapy-seekers in India do not see different forms of therapy and their different conceptions of illness as mutually exclusive or contradictory.[14]

I cannot help but think that the issue of high educational achievement and the lack of commensurate jobs in Kerala, which I believe relates to the state's high suicide rate (Halliburton 1998), may have implications for Abdul-Rahman's situation. Abdul-Rahman had completed his Secondary School Leaving Certificate, which should raise his prospects of employment beyond low-paid manual labor positions. Although he comes across as a very intelligent person, he did not do a Pre-Degree Certificate (PDC) that would have qualified him for college entry. It is probably frustrating for him to work delivering newspapers, and this experience may be compounded by his having returned from the Gulf under emotional duress rather than as the heroic "Gulfan" whose money and prestige make him a "man about town" (Osella and Osella 2000b: 123) and help him "progress along a culturally idealized trajectory towards mature manhood" (118).

It is probably Abdul-Rahman's active mind, turned inward and under distress, that contributes to the awkward character of his speech. Biju and I were constantly tested in trying to interpret and translate his remarks. Abdul-Rahman's narrative style gave the impression of someone who was thinking rapidly while trying to speak. What he said seemed to have many meanings, and also betrayed a sense of indecisiveness, uncertainty and frustration. We did not receive any response to our letter, sent seven months after this interview, requesting a follow-up meeting. I hope Abdul-Rahman found fulfilling work or at least a way to get some satisfying rest and a sense of focus.

Rajendran and His Wife: The Clerk Who Skipped Work

Kavitha and I interviewed Rajendran and his wife at a private allopathic psychiatric hospital in Trivandrum where Rajendran was receiving treatment. Rajendran is a 47-year-old, university-educated, Hindu man who works at a bank as a senior clerk. Rajendran does not feel that anything is wrong with him, although his wife and son brought him to this hospital out of concern that he wasn't sleeping or eating normally. He had also missed work and had taken to writing strange things.

After learning how Rajendran rose from cashier to become senior clerk over his 24-year career at the same bank, Kavitha asked him about his educational qualifications:

Kavitha: Until what level have you studied? Have you done "degree" [bachelor's degree] and all?

Rajendran: Yes. After completing my "degree course," I did not attempt the exam. But I have a feeling that someone wrote the exam using my number because when I wrote the exam the second time and passed, the result was "withheld."

Kavitha: I see.

Rajendran: At that time, I couldn't inquire about it in the university. I was busy. After that, I have been without a "degree." I did not write the exam in March [many years ago]. In March, some friends wrote it for me. After that, I wrote, but did not "pass" the exam. I completed "degree" studies. I did "maths main" for my "degree."

People's educational histories are major topics of discussion in Kerala, and this is a relatively modest and concise answer to a question about educational achievements. Some younger male informants we met spoke for fifteen minutes or more explaining how they did on each exam on each attempt and where they ranked in their class at different stages. The educational pressure in Kerala begins in elementary school when students are expected to study three languages and several disciplinary subjects, and pass exams in these areas. Although most people do not study beyond secondary school, high school and university enrollment have increased dramatically in the last few decades.[15]

We then changed the topic of conversation to Rajendran's reason for admission to this psychiatric facility, and he explained that he was unaware of any problem that might be afflicting him:

On March 31, we had to do some "overtime" work on "government treasury bills." So I was preparing for that, but in the end no one asked me to work "overtime." So I thought that was good and went home and took rest. Working overtime will be a "strain" on our body and mind. After that, I had to go back to the bank on the second, but I was tired so I couldn't. My wife thought that I was doing it intentionally. I hadn't gone to work for overtime, and on the third they took me here. I don't know what complaint they have about me. I don't know what there is to "complain" about. I did not go to work on the second. That's all.

When we asked whether Rajendran had had any problems in the past, he explained that he saw a doctor in 1983 for blurry vision, but provided an unusual explanation of the situation:

One day in '83, I slept late. The next morning . . . Not only that, I slept very late. I heard a commotion. I live next to Engineering College. I heard some girls yelling from the Engineering College compound. I thought of going there with my wife. I wanted to go there with weapons and try to help them. When I thought of this, everyone got up and asked me not to leave the house. So both of us went to sleep, but I couldn't sleep. That day, at 10 o'clock when I counted cash, I couldn't see the notes clearly. So I gave the charge to another person. I was the only person doing cash so I gave the charge to another clerk and left.

Like his current situation, this earlier problem had some relation to work, to leaving his office. A little later, Rajendran reasserted, "I don't have any illness. On the second, because I was late, I didn't go." He said that the following day he was ready to go to work when his son said he needed Rajendran to accompany him to inquire about getting admission to a tutorial program to help with his studies. This, however, turned out to be a ruse by his wife and son to bring him to the psychiatric hospital.

When we asked what other remedies he had sought for his problem, he told us that 11 years earlier he saw an astrologer who told him he had not done anything wrong that might have caused his difficulties. Rajendran also explained that he has been taking over-the-counter ayurvedic medicines including *chandanadi* oil to help him sleep and *brahmi*, the treatment for mental strengthening used by ayurvedic doctors, Chottanikkara temple officials and some Muslim priests. We returned to the topic of Rajendran's current illness, at which point his wife took over and spoke on his behalf for the remainder of the interview:

Kavitha: What is the reason you are here now?

Rajendran's Wife: We came because he is not getting enough sleep. He won't sleep before 2 am, and won't eat any food. He will always watch me serving the food and will eat only if he likes it. He is suspicious of whether the food is clean, and if he doesn't like it he won't eat it. If he likes it, he will eat only a little. He won't eat anything. Now, after coming here, he is looking healthy. Before that, he was too thin.

Kavitha: Is that the reason for coming here?

Rajendran's Wife: Yes. He is not sleeping. And we can't read what he writes. There will be no sense to it.

Kavitha: And when he talks?

Rajendran's Wife: There is no problem when he talks. He speaks well. When he writes, we can't understand anything. So we thought, how can this be happening? He will make noises with his pen by hitting it on the paper. When we ask why he is doing this, he will say that he is trying to destroy "bombs" and is listening for their sound.

Kavitha: Is it the first time he is having this sight problem?

Rajendran's Wife: Yes. He is working in a bank. When he goes for his work, he complains that someone is shining a light in his eyes so he can't work. Then he says, "Someone is shooting at me and small pellets are in my body." He says things like this.

Rajendran's wife reiterated her concern about her husband not eating and becoming thin later in our interview. Suspicion about food being unclean or poisoned was seen in other male informants. One complained that his wife was intentionally making bad food and not serving meals at the right time. Problems related to food—refusing to eat, eating little, eating slowly and being suspicious of food—were often reported by patients and their relatives. Although the eating problems mentioned here are frequently seen among people suffering mental distress in Kerala, cases of anorexia and obesity are extremely rare in this setting according to mental health practitioners and my own observations of patients.

Rajendran's wife explained that the first time Rajendran's problems emerged, he was brought to the psychiatric hospital where he is now receiving treatment. "Then," his wife recalled, "he reduced the medicine by himself and like that stopped taking it. On his own, without the doctor's approval, he said he is not ill and stopped taking medicine. When he stopped taking medicine, the problem came back." About two years ago, Rajendran's wife took him to see Father M., a church minister and psychiatrist. Like Sreedevi's mother, who learned about ayurvedic psychiatric specialists from a newspaper, Rajendran's wife read about Father M. in *Mangalam*, a popular magazine. Father M. hypnotized Rajendran and gave him medicine. "He got lots of change, lots of relief from there," his wife recalled. As with other patients who crossed religious lines in pursuit of a therapy that will give relief, Rajendran and his wife are Hindu, but this did not inhibit them from seeking therapy from a Christian practitioner.

When asked to explain how Rajendran's problems started, his wife traced their origin to the death of his father with whom he and his wife had a special relationship:

The first time this happened is when his father died. He was very fond of his father. He married me without his family's permission. He is my cousin. My uncle's son. So his father and mother did not approve. I don't have enough education. I studied only until 7th [year of schooling]. So his family didn't like it, but we got married. My family also did not like the idea. So we got married out of love. So we don't go see our family. Only his father came to us and loved us even after our marriage. He died after we had three children. So when his father died he [Rajendran] probably thought that he did not have anyone to love, that he lost his love. So then his father died, and when they took his body he [Rajendran] too was taken to Medical College hospital. He was unconscious so his friends took him. They [the doctors] wrote that this was mental and gave

treatment for that. His friends did not show that [probably referring to a diagnosis of mental illness written in Rajendran's records or in a prescription] to us
or anyone. If he had done something, if he had taken medicine continuously, it
wouldn't have been like this.

Despite the trauma of his father dying, there was no indication of Rajendran
receiving any treatment other than medications. Rajendran's wife meanwhile
asserts her belief in a pharmaceutical solution to her husband's problems. At
the end of the interview, Rajendran's wife said she believes he has improved
during his stay at this hospital, and she heard he may be released soon:

Kavitha: When will he go from here, get improvement and leave here?

Rajendran's Wife: Doctor did not say anything about that. The nurse said that
we can go on this Sunday. Maybe we can go on Sunday.

Kavitha: Do you believe that this problem won't come again? Or, if it does, will
you come here, or . . .?

Rajendran's Wife: We will only come here. We won't go anywhere else.

Rajendran's wife did not rule out the possibility of Rajendran's problem
returning, but, as opposed to Abdul-Rahman who says he is open to using
any kind of therapy to get relief, she affirms an allegiance to this hospital.
Yet Rajendran was continuing to take ayurvedic medications to treat himself,
indicating that the boundaries between medical categories are somewhat fluid
for this couple. We did not see Rajendran again, and were unable to arrange
a follow-up interview with him. I hope that Rajendran and his family have
found relief, or at least a way to live with his problems.

Lakshmi: The Gulf Wife, Blessed by Devi

Lakshmi is a 26-year-old woman who is not employed and whose husband is
in Saudi Arabia doing manual labor. When Biju and I met Lakshmi, she and
several relatives were staying at Chottanikkara temple on one of the visits they
regularly undertake for prayer and the maintenance of Lakshmi's health.
  We interviewed Lakshmi and her relatives in their room at the temple guest
lodge, where Biju and I were also staying. Lakshmi's relatives did not speak
during the interview, but Rajan, the young man who works at the temple lodge
whose own experiences with possession were presented in Chapter 2, also

attended and made comments. Rajan got to know most of the patient-devotees who were staying at the lodge, and he helped arrange some of our interviews.

One of the first things we learned about Lakshmi was that she had gone pretty far in her studies. She completed her PDC which makes her eligible to apply to a university, but she did not have a job and was not attending school, a gap between educational achievement and employment that is encountered by many women in Kerala (Forero-Peña 2004).

When we asked Lakshmi what problem she was seeking relief from in coming to Chottanikkara temple, she explained:

I had illness all over my body. Even when I took medicine I did not get any better. After that, we went to a *bhajanamatham* [a religious center] where one can
get Amma's [Devi, the goddess] blessings [*anugraham*]. When we went to the
place where you receive the blessing, we came to know through Amma that this
illness keeps on coming because we have this *dōsham* [astrological sign/fault].
After that, we came here for *bhajana* [worship through singing]. Just one worship made it so that we didn't need to go to a hospital.

Biju: What type of illnesses did you have?

Rajan: You spoke about many serious *asvasthatakal* [uneasinesses/discomforts]?

Lakshmi: Yes, there was *asvasthata*, always a fever, chronic fever, headache all the
time. Pain all over the body.

Here Lakshmi explains that her distress is expressed through the body. Although I argue later that people in Kerala draw a clear distinction between mind and body and conceive of certain behavioral problems as "mental ill-nesses" (*manasika rogam*), many people at religious and psychiatric healing centers expressed emotional troubles somatically, through the body. Categorizing or locating "distress" in the person is complex. It can originate in personal, social, family or work problems and manifest as symptoms or suffering that is "mental," "emotional," "physical" or "spiritual"—or any or all of these at the same time. Lakshmi's explanation of the cause of her problem similarly defies easy classification in this kind of analytic, medical, secular terminology. She recalls that she learned from Amma that her illness is caused by a *dōsham*, a bad sign, a sin or bad karma, with which she was born. This problem emerged six years ago at which time Lakshmi saw an allopathic doctor. Regarding her experience with allopathy, Lakshmi said, "I will get relief [*āśvāsam*], but when I come home, it will start again." Lakshmi also began visiting Chottanikkara six years ago, and she describes her experience there with some enthusiasm:

I have been coming to Chottanikkara for the last six years now. I came here because of the *chaitanyam* [power/consciousness] and blessing of the Devi [the goddess] at Chottanikkara. I started sitting for worship. From then until now, I haven't been to the "hospital." I have no problem at all. I came here, and Devi changed everything in me. So I have been getting *aiśvaryam* [wealth/glory] and *abhivriddhi* [prosperity] continuously. Because of that blessing, I will be here forever.

When someone depicts their experiences in healing or medical treatment, we do not expect exuberant descriptions. The stories of "healing" encountered in Kerala were not usually exuberant and often recalled incremental changes or complete remediation, for the time being, but "healing" can involve something more. What some people in Kerala said they accomplished through healing was not just a ridding or reduction of a problem but, as Lakshmi describes here, an attainment of a state that is somehow higher and more vibrant than one's original, pre-illness state. Not only does Lakshmi say she no longer has a problem, she claims to have gained "prosperity" and the "blessing" of Devi. While patients of allopathy say that they got good "relief" or became "completely healthy," a number of informants who used religious therapy recalled their experience with enthusiasm and nostalgia and described undergoing a positive transformation. Like allopathic patients, ayurvedic patients generally spoke of returning to a state of health or simply getting some relief, although a few say they attained an enhanced state of health. When Lakshmi says "I will be here forever," she is expressing her intention to keep returning to Chottanikkara, or she may simply mean she will always feel connected to the temple in some way. Lakshmi lives in a neighboring district of Kerala, and her family visits Chottanikkara once a month. Lakshmi recalled the first time she encountered Devi at Chottanikkara:

The first time I saw Devi, I had come here before. I came, and I left after only doing *tozhuka* [adoring the deity with hands together at the chest in traditional *namaskāram* greeting pose]. I had not sat for worship like this. The first time I came here to sit for worship, many wonders were worked on me. The reason is, first, people came here with the same illnesses. I did not understand what it was. After some time, when we sat there, it felt like something was leaving our body. It cured/changed [*māri*] all our uneasiness. We were changing in our selves.[16]

Then Rajan joined the conversation to ask Lakshmi about the first time she became possessed:

Rajan: How was it when you "first" got possessed [*tullāl*]?

Lakshmi: The "first" time I got possessed, I felt like I was being tied up.

Biju: Like you were tied up?

Lakshmi: Like being chained at the legs, unable to walk.

Biju: Do you feel like someone is coming to "attack" you? Like someone is "attacking" you from behind?

(Brief conversation between Murphy and Biju.)

Lakshmi: When we do that, we will feel each thing inside us, inside our mind like each thing working on us. That is, whether we do some prayer or when we come to do something else, without obstacles, we . . . When some obstacle comes, we make some promise [to Devi]: that after getting beyond that obstacle, we will come back. Sometimes, we will not be able to move our tongue. Finally, we will be unable to talk. Then when we do offerings, we will be free from that.

Biju: Do you have consciousness [*bōdham*] during possession [*tullāl*]? Consciousness [*bōdham*]?

Lakshmi: No.

Biju: Do you have [literally, "see"] consciousness inside [*ullil bōdham kānumō*] ?

Lakshmi: Inside the inside, there will be consciousness [*ullinte ullil bōdham kānum*]. The reason is . . . but there is no outside. There is a feeling that something is inside.

Biju: No consciousness [*bōdham*] on the outside, right?

Lakshmi: No consciousness [*bōdhamilla*].

In this exchange, Lakshmi is saying that during possession, her normal state of consciousness is gone ("there is no outside"), but at some, deep or subtle level ("inside the inside") she is aware of what is happening. This discussion about possession turns on the idiom *bōdham* "consciousness," one of several principle modes of experience in the local phenomenology—the culturally and historically shaped way of dividing up and orienting experience—Biju and Lakshmi are engaging with. In Chapter 4 we will see that people in Kerala experience problems of distress in terms of a variety of states that form a continuum from the tangible body to the intangible *ātman* or true self. *Bōdham* lies toward the less tangible—and more highly valued—end of this continuum. Lakshmi's affliction seems to have affected her whole person. Earlier, she described how she experienced problems as discomforts in the body, and here she expresses her affliction in terms of subtly distinct levels of consciousness and a change in the self.

As our conversation continued, we learned more about the *dōsham* that caused Lakshmi's troubles:

Biju: What do you think is the cause of your problem? You have some problems and all, "okay"? You had a problem earlier, right? What do you think is the reason for that problem?

Lakshmi: *Sarppadōsham* [snake *dōsham*/sign].

Biju: *Sarppadōsham*? How did you learn about s*arppadōsham*?

Lakshmi: How I learned it was when we were getting possessed. At that time, it comes to us. We will know it clearly.

Sarppadōsham is an inauspicious sign, and someone born with this *dōsham* is expected to encounter adversity. Western academic and popular representations of *karma* and Indian astrology give the impression of a belief in an irreversible fate that must be passively accepted. Karma and astrological signs, however, are merely part of a complex interplay of divine and human forces that shape action and destiny. Divine and human actions can change the impact of astrological signs, and it appears that for Lakshmi the effects of *sarppadōsham* have been superseded with help from Devi.

Finally, we learned that Lakshmi married seven years ago, and for the last five years her husband has been working in the Persian Gulf and is able to visit home only sporadically. Such "Gulf marriages," as they are known in Kerala, was the topic of the Master's thesis in psychology that my assistant Kavitha completed at the University of Kerala. Kavitha examined mental health among women in Gulf marriages and found that Gulf wives were more depressed and had more "maladjustment traits" than women whose husbands were living in Kerala. Yet the two groups showed no difference in "stress" and "mental health status." Additionally, Gulf wives who were not working suffered greater stress than those who were employed (Kavitha 1996).[17] These "Gulf marriage" adversities must weigh heavily on Lakshmi who remains unemployed despite having good educational qualifications. Still, she sounds confident that Devi will help her keep her problems at bay and maintain the auspicious state she feels she has achieved.

Six months after this interview, we sent follow-up questions by mail to learn of any changes in Lakshmi's condition and therapy-seeking practices. We conducted in-person, follow-up interviews with informants who lived near Trivandrum District, where Kavitha, Biju and I resided, but informants who lived in more distant regions of Kerala, such as Lakshmi, were asked to respond to written questions sent by mail. Whereas it would not be practical to follow up such informants in other parts of India (unless one was doing an epidemiological study with a large number of researchers), Kerala's near-total literacy makes it possible to at least seek written responses from patients who live in other regions of the state. An unidentified male, most likely a family member writing on Lakshmi's behalf, gave us the following responses to our follow-up inquiry:

1) How do you feel at present? Have you experienced any improvement or decline in your condition?

She is feeling good. She has experienced improvement.[18]

2) What treatment have you been using since we last spoke with you (about 6 months ago)?

She is taking treatment now.

3) How many times have you been to Chottanikkara temple since we last spoke with you?

Each month we are going to Chottanikkara. In addition to that, we are doing two or three days *bhajana* [devotional singing].

4) Do you have any symptoms you did not notice before (since we last met)?

No.

5) Do you have any new ideas about the cause of your illness? Please explain what you believe to be the cause of your illness.

Now there is no problem.

6) If your problems are still continuing, do you have any specific plan to get over this illness?

There is no problem, but if anything should arise, we have faith that we can solve the problem by *bhakti* [devotion].

7) If your problems are still continuing, when do you believe these problems will be over?

[no answer]

8) Please give us any additional comments you feel we should know.

If you want to know more details, please contact this address.

We are told that, six months after our original interview, Lakshmi is doing well, and there is confidence that any further problems can be resolved through engaging in devotional practices and visiting Chottanikkara. As reflected in this fortuitous assessment of Lakshmi's condition, informants using religious therapies reported the greatest degree of improvement in our follow-up interviews and questionnaires although their self-prognoses were only slightly better than those of patients who were using allopathy or ayurveda.[19]

Hanifa and His Wife: Relieving "Tension" at Beemapalli

Hanifa and his wife had been staying at Beemapalli and seeking relief for Hanifa's problems for a year and a half when Kavitha and I met them. Hanifa is a 30-year-old Muslim man from Trivandrum District who worked for five years as a janitor in the Persian Gulf. Less educated than most of the patients profiled in this chapter—although still well-educated by the standards of most other Indian states—Hanifa remained in school through the 10th standard but then failed the exam for the Secondary School Leaving Certificate. While in the Gulf, Hanifa developed psychological problems—"tension" he and his wife later called them using the English term—which led him to resign from his job and return home. Hanifa described for us the nature of his problem and the treatment he received from an allopathic psychiatrist:

> Sleeplessness was one problem, and for that he would give medicine to be taken at night. I should take pills at night, and get up only in the morning. He said not to take that medicine in the morning. He will give me the prescription, and I will get it from medical shop. Then he asks me to meet him next "term," and then I will go and consult him. He will again give some prescription for medicine and we will buy it and it will go on like that "continuously."

Like Abdul-Rahman, Hanifa's recollection of his allopathic treatment focuses on medication, affirming Nunley's (1996) observation that psychiatric patients in India associate allopathic therapy primarily with the administration of drugs. Although he saw this psychiatrist in his private practice, where therapists normally have more time to engage in talk therapy, Hanifa did not give any indication that he received any psychotherapy or counseling. We then inquired whether he had any difficulties other than sleeplessness, and he explained, "Something like a 'tension' has come," using the English-language idiom that Mary also invoked.

After seeing the allopathic psychiatrist, Hanifa sought therapy from a clinical psychologist for one month. Hanifa and his wife had also been coming to Beemapalli since the onset of Hanifa's "tension:"

> Hanifa's Wife: Right from when this problem started, we used to come here once a week.

> Kavitha: Here.

> Hanifa's Wife: After that, for one and a half years we have been staying here. We have to stay here for five more months. There is a lot of change after coming here.

> Hanifa: After we married, I got a son. He's five years old.

> Kavitha: Yeah, I saw him.

> Hanifa's Wife: This "tension" began when he was working in the Gulf. So he resigned from the job and came back. Then his father's death. Then there was some problem. After that the business also was not beneficial and we lost everything. Then there was a financial problem also.

Hanifa's problems were compounded by the death of his father and financial difficulties he and his wife encountered after his return from the Gulf. His wife says here that coming to Beemapalli has brought him "a lot of change," although the allopathic psychological and psychiatric treatment that partially overlaps this period may have contributed to this improvement. We asked Hanifa's wife if they were still continuing allopathic treatment:

> Kavitha: Are you taking allopathic medicine now?

> Hanifa's Wife: No, no.

> Kavitha: Now he is not taking any medicine.

> Murphy: Now it is finished.

> Hanifa's Wife: Now that he is not taking medicine, there is a lot of improvement. When he was taking medicine, he had memory problems [lit. reduction: *kuravu*].

We later asked Hanifa's wife whether it was these memory problems that led them to discontinue allopathic care:

Kavitha: Was it because of memory problems that you stopped, or . . .?

Hanifa's Wife: Yeah, because of memory problems and a lot of "tension." Thinking, and he was like this. So we changed. Now there is relief after coming here. After he came here, he sleeps without taking medicine. Before this he wouldn't sleep even after taking two pills.

Our discussion about medications with Hanifa's wife will be revisited in Chapter 5 in considering how "pleasant" it is to undergo treatment in these different systems of healing. Hanifa is one of several patients who left allopathic psychiatric treatment because they did not like the effects of medications. Hanifa has been living at Beemapalli where his wife says he gets "relief" and can sleep, which is reminiscent of other people we spoke with who appeared to have found a way to cope with intractable or recurring problems, not by pursuing medical solutions but by living with their problems in a "pleasant" therapeutic environment—that is, in an environment that is aesthetically engaging and where undergoing therapeutic practices, the process of therapy itself and not just the effect therapy aims to generate, is therapeutic. In Hanifa's case, his problem is not resolved or cured, but he gets some relief by residing in the aesthetically and spiritually engaging environment of Beemapalli mosque.

Allopathy was the most common form of therapy that people suffering mental afflictions used before coming to Beemapalli, but many had also tried ayurveda, *mantravādam* (sorcery), homeopathy, and visiting temples before resorting to the mosque to find relief.

As our interview continued, we asked if Hanifa had received any kind of psychotherapy:

Kavitha: Did the "doctors" give you "counseling"?

Hanifa: What does that mean?

Kavitha: Did they talk to you for a long time to get everything in your mind?

Hanifa: Yes, they will ask me some questions.

Kavitha: They will talk for some time, and after that do you get any "relief?"

Hanifa: "Are you sleeping well?" They will ask me if I have enough sleep now. Then they will ask me if I can hear some voices talking to me. Only when I take medicine I will sleep. Without that I can't sleep, even in the daytime. They told me to continue the medicine.

Hanifa reveals his unfamiliarity with counseling and psychotherapy and recalls only diagnostic questions doctors had asked him. He concludes his response with a return to the topic of medication.

We resumed discussing Hanifa's troubles, and his wife told us that he was under tension in the Gulf partly because of financial concerns. Like many migrant workers from India, he had to borrow a large sum of money to obtain a plane ticket, visa and work permit at a time when he and his family were not economically secure. Now they are doing better financially, according to Hanifa's wife, who then offered further details about his troubles:

Since he came back, if we ask him anything, he will get *veprālam* [confusion, worry] and will run off. He will run off without telling anyone. When we look for him, he won't be in the house. He began to spend all of our money. So then for some time we thought it might be *kaivisham* [a mysterious poison] or *śeyittān* [a spirit]. So we were looking into that.

Kavitha: Did you do any *pūja* [worship, ritual] for that?

Hanifa's Wife: We didn't do a lot of that. His sister is educated so they consulted a doctor. There was no relief with that. Only when we came here to this mosque was there any change [*māttam*].

Again, Hanifa's wife emphasized that Hanifa's problem improved only at Beemapalli mosque. She then told us that they had tried *pūjas* (worships and rituals that can have a Hindu connotation) to counter *kshudram* (sorcery) in case Hanifa's troubles are caused by *kaivisham* or a *śeyittān*, as his wife suspected. These efforts, however, did not improve Hanifa's condition.

Hanifa's wife told us earlier that they had to remain in Beemapalli only five more months for Hanifa to get relief. Toward the end of the interview, when we asked her to explain how she knew this, she recalled that Umma [the woman who is entombed at Beemapalli] revealed this in a dream:

We will dream about it, and in the dream we will be given medicines, an "operation" and all. If we dream that we are going home, we can go home. We dreamt of being here until the flag hoisting [the annual festival at the mosque]. After that we can go.

Biju, Kavitha and I returned to Beemapalli several times and conducted follow-up interviews with informants we saw on the mosque grounds, but we did not meet Hanifa and his wife again. It is possible we simply did not notice them among the many people who circulate through the mosque every day. It is my hope that Hanifa and his wife completed their five months, got some "change," and returned home.

Features of everyday life, social practices and transnational influences in Kerala arise in these conversations with people suffering mental distress. Educational achievement and marriage choice were significant concerns for virtually every person presented here. From Rajendran, we got a taste of how people in Kerala discuss their educational qualifications and the exams they passed or failed. Sreedevi's mother, herself a school teacher, expressed her concern about her daughter's loss of interest in studies. Sreedevi also revealed, along with Mary, concerns and anxieties about marriage prospects and the nature of married life. Marriage concerns were encountered in Rajendran's story as well, especially in relation to the death of his father, the one person who supported Rajendran and his wife in a marriage that was condemned by other members of their families.

The trials and (mis)fortunes of Persian Gulf migration also affected the economic and mental stability of several of these patients. Abdul-Rahman and Hanifa associated the development of their mental distress with their experiences in and early return from the Gulf. Lakshmi's husband, meanwhile, has been working in the Gulf for several years, and although she did not explicitly connect her problems to this situation, the fact that she has to remain at home, unemployed and unable to see her husband may well contribute to her mental distress.

We also saw evidence of the dissemination of knowledge about health and healing through the popular press in Kerala in the stories of these individuals and their families. Sreedevi's mother learned about ayurvedic psychiatry through the newspaper, and Rajendran's wife took her husband to see a church minister-psychiatrist whom she read about in a popular magazine. Allopathic psychiatric and psychological views are more often represented in the media. Although as we know from the testimony of Sreedevi's mother and Rajendran's wife that allopathic discourse about mental health has not become hegemonic, we will see later how allopathic idioms, such as the "tension" reported by Hanifa, are creating new hybrid discourses of illness.

These patient narratives also reveal some of the variety of Malayalam terms used to describe what one accomplishes through therapy, including the forms of the verb *māruka* ("to change", *mātti, māri, mārum*), *vyatyāsam* ("difference" in a positive sense, improvement), *kuravu* ("decline" or "lessening" of negative symptoms), *āśvāsam* ("relief"), *aiśvaryam* ("wealth/glory") and *abhivriddhi* ("prosperity"). None of these terms has quite the same meaning as "cure," and the case of Hanifa, who finds relief by residing for periods of time at Beemapalli mosque, presents an example of a way of coping with an illness problem that is not captured by the allopathic/English language ideal of curing. Thus people's illness experiences in Kerala give us a variety of ways of thinking about the goals of healing and the dispensation of illness, some of which challenge the understanding of healing or curing as a return to an original pre-illness state or a simple absence of illness.

Finally, Lakshmi parses the different types of consciousness she experiences during possession while Sreedevi and Mary clearly identify their problems as occurring in the realm of *manas* ("mind"), providing hints of a construction of phenomenological experience that is neither "embodied" nor a case of mind-body dualism.

Notes

1. Privileging the interior, individual self as somehow more authentic is likely to be problematic in North American and European societies as well—see Kusserow (1996, 1999) on the socially embedded self in the United States and Battaglia (1995), who claims the self is "a reification continually defeated by mutable entanglements with other subjects' histories, experience, self-representations" (2).
2. This and all other quotes from informants are translated from Malayalam, although words in quotation marks occurred in English in the original. In order to preserve readability, not all English language terms are indicated by quotes in all interviews. Certain frequently used English terms that have become part of everyday speech in Malayalam, such as "doctor," "hospital" or names of medications are not highlighted.
3. Approximately 15% of people in Kerala pass SSLC, and this is one of the highest rates in India (National Family Health Survey—Kerala 1995: 33, 189).
4. National Family Health Survey—India (1995: 53).
5. The drug names the informants indicate are brand names, not generic names. The same psychiatric drugs that are available in the United States are made by Indian pharmaceutical companies and are marketed under brand names different from those in the U.S. Hexidol, which Sreedevi's mother mentions here, is the brand name of a commonly prescribed antipsychotic. It is a combination of haloperidol and benzhexol hydrocholoride.
6. Romanucci-Ross (1969), Young (1981) and Sharp (1994).
7. On the availability of allopathic care in Kerala, see Panikar and Soman (1984) and Nirmala (1997).
8. An online encyclopedia by an Indian botanical research institute lists 17 different species that are locally referred to as "raktapushpa" in India (Foundation for the Revitalization of Local Health Traditions 2006). A newly discovered species of

Humboldtia brunonis in Kerala was named *Humboldtia brunonis raktapushpa* by researchers who identified the plant because of the plant's red flowers (Udayan, Tushar and George 2007). The researchers who identified this species—which was already known to the local community where it was found—were working for the Centre for Medicinal Plants Research of the Arya Vaidya Sala, the large ayurvedic pharmaceutical manufacturer and research center in Kottakkal discussed in Chapter 2. This example hints at a common interest in plants in ayurveda and religious healing in Kerala. Although the understanding may be ritual-symbolic in one realm and physiological in the other, there is occasional overlap as in the case of the ayurvedic medicine *brahmi*, which is given to the afflicted at Chottanikkara. The ingestion of plants may, in turn, have implications that are simultaneously physiological, ritualistic and symbolic.

9. English words commonly appear in Malayalam discourse, but using the English word "change" rather than some form of *māruka* is somewhat unusual. As a schoolteacher, Sreedevi's mother would be expected to have some proficiency in English, and she may have been trying to impress me and Biju or make her story easier for me to follow.

10. A priest or pastor—from a Malayalam word *achchan* that translates as "father" and refers to a male cleric of any Christian denomination.

11. With a national average of 9.9 suicides per 100,000 people in India in the 1990s, Kerala had an astonishingly high suicide rate of 28 per 100,000, the highest of any Indian state and almost twice as high as the state with the second highest rate (National Crime Records Bureau 1994: 58). Kerala's high suicide rate seems to relate to a gap between high educational attainment and the lack of commensurate jobs and possibly other social processes involved in secularization and "modernization" in the state (Halliburton 1998).

12. Saith (1992: 114–115), Thomas Isaac (1997), *The Hindu* (April 10, 1997) and Waldman (2003).

13. As Osella and Osella observe, "In popular films and plays, the returning *gulfan* is invariably portrayed arriving by taxi from the airport, the car loaded with boxes and parcels. He wears a designer shirt, white trousers and the latest sports shoes. He smokes *foreign* cigarettes and wears Ray-Ban sunglasses. . . . He is a man about town . . . He pays very large dowries for the marriage of his sisters, and, when he marries, receives a large dowry" (2000b: 123).

14. See Carstairs and Kapur (1976: 66), Nichter (1981: 5) and Weiss et al. (1986: 380).

15. E. T. Mathew observed that from the foundation of the state of Kerala in 1956 until 1990–91, enrollment has increased 77% in primary education, 591% in secondary education, and 1,518% at university level (1997: 102).

16. In the last three lines of this passage, Lakshmi is using the inclusive form of "we" and "our" here (*nammal/nammalute*) in which the person or persons being addressed is included in the "we" (literally, "our body" here means the body of Lakshmi, Biju and everyone she is speaking to, as if they collectively possessed a single body, and she is describing an experience where her interlocutors were not present). The inclusive "we" in Malayalam establishes a solidarity between speaker and listener and is characteristic of the socially embedded "self" that is shaped by everyday discourses and practices in Kerala.

17. Also, a study by Gulati (1983) claimed that the incidence of mental illness was higher in areas of Kerala that had the highest rates of Gulf migration.

18. Although the original Malayalam responses are subjectless, and the verb does not indicate who the speaker is, I added "she" to make the response intelligible in English. As the subjectless construction in Malayalam may indicate the use of a relational sense of self or a social group as the subject, this response may be additionally understood to attest to the family having experienced improvement and relief.

19. For further analysis of effectiveness and outcome for patients of these three therapies, see Halliburton (2004).

4

⌘

EXPERIENCING THE WORLD FROM BODY TO *ĀTMAN*

In the 1990s, researchers in anthropology and other fields became enthralled with the possibility of transcending mind-body dualism. The modern assumption that illness and other experiences are either of the mind or of the body had become dissatisfying to many. Mind-body dualism was exposed as a Western construct first articulated in the work of Descartes, and many non-Western cultures offered alternative approaches that revealed the intertwining of body and mind, emotion and cognition and other dualities. This chapter complicates this story, and evokes the particular, localized variety of ways people attend to sensory and phenomenological experience.

While academic studies of the body do provide an important critique of earlier research that had considered experience in mentalistic and representational terms and through the assumptions of Western mind-body dualism, there has developed a tendency to use this analytic corrective to depict non-Western cultures as grounding experience in the body and as lacking a phenomenological orientation that distinguishes mind from body. In other words, the exotic Other has come to serve as the aesthetic, earthly antidote to a West that was imagined as overly cerebral and disembodied. "Mental" patients and possessed people in Kerala reveal a variety of tangible and intangible modes of experience that include distinctions between mind and body yet portray an orientation to experience—or a "phenomenology," as I call such orientations—that differs from Western mind-body dualism. At the outset of this study, I claimed that phenomenological experience is to some degree locally constructed. Here,

I show how people I met in Kerala mediate experience through a particular phenomenological orientation consisting of aspects of the person—including *śarīram* (body), *manas* (mind), *bōdham* (consciousness) and *ātman* (true self/ soul)—that lie along a continuum of increasing intangibility ranging from the gross, tangible body to the abstract and disembodied *ātman*.

Rather than focusing on the body or examples of mind-body transcendence, it would be more productive for researchers to examine local, culturally and historically shaped phenomenologies which are constellations of various parts of the person that mediate people's experience of the world. One may still wish to consider the role of the body in a social setting, but developing an understanding of local phenomenology—which may be shaped by trans-local ideologies and practices—provides an indispensable context for assessing the status and role of the body and embodied experience. This exploration into Kerala phenomenology gives us a more complete depiction of the experience of people suffering "mental" distress and provides insights into universal and variable features of human experience.

Focusing on the Body

Research on the body and embodiment in anthropology and other disciplines has been prolific in the last two decades. Perhaps analogous to the tendency for anthropologists to assume the distant Other to be living in a remote time, the excitement about finding alternatives to the allegedly mentalistic West has led researchers to locate the Other more firmly in the body.[1] Ethnographers have asserted that peoples in New Guinea locate emotion and moral issues in the heart or the skin (Strathern 1996), that "consciousness . . . cannot be disembodied," sorcery is always "body seeking" in Sri Lanka (Kapferer 1997: 44) and that "[t]he Yaka [of Zaire] perceive of the body as the pivotal point from which the subject gradually develops a sense of identity" (Devisch 1993: 139). People in Kerala, however, do not seem to experience things this way. They do to some degree live through the body, but they are also emphatically concerned with the mind, with "consciousness," which is distinct from the mind, and with the intangible self.

Ethnographic studies of the body and embodiment focus primarily on people outside Europe or North America. Work on the body the United States has focused on non-Western immigrant groups, while research on Latin America looks to pre-Hispanic culture for evidence of embodied modes of experience. When one also considers that much of the contemporary research on the body in Western culture outside of anthropology focuses on women and oppressed ethnic groups and that some have associated expressing suffering through the body with low socioeconomic position, one gets the impression that it is people who have less access to power that locate experience more firmly in the body or transcend mind-body dualism.[2] In particular, distress that is expressed in the form of emotional or mental problems in the Western middle class world is allegedly expressed through physical, somatic symptoms elsewhere.[3] In contrast to these studies, the examples of supra-somatic expressions—concerns about consciousness and the less tangible parts of the person—I observed in Kerala cut across class, gender and religious lines.

Those who focus on social suffering (Kleinman and Kleinman 1995; Kleinman, Das and Lock 1997) and personhood (Pollock 1996) offer the potential for analyses of experience that do not overindulge the body and consider a diversity of experiential conditions. Social suffering includes the notion of illness, but is broader, taking into account the mental, bodily and indeterminate other expressions of distress that stem from social pressure ranging from stress to "nerves" to political violence. Also, particular ethnographies, such as Robert Desjarlais' (1997) depiction of the lives of the homeless in Boston and Lawrence Cohen's (1998) analysis of aging in India, investigate embodiment and experience without falling into the mentally-oriented Westerner-embodied Other dichotomy. Desjarlais' definition of experience as "a historically and culturally constituted process predicated on certain ways of being in the world" (1997:13) resembles my characterization of local phenomenologies. We need to understand that the person and her engagement with the world are defined not by dichotomies but by fine-tuned, localized orientations to experience.

Johnathan Parry (1989) explains that his ethnographic material on the dispensation of the body at death in Banaras, in north India, and informants' explanations of the conditions of birth and rebirth show a monistic relation between body, mind and soul—that the food one consumes and one's thoughts can alter one's body and bio-moral substance and that the state of the body reveals the state of the soul. Parry claims his material also reveals evidence of a dualism of matter and spirit: that mind is more important than body for salvation (512). Parry suggests one could interpret these explanations as exhibiting characteristics of both monism and dualism regarding matters of material and spirit. In other words, material substance and spirit are both integrated and yet distinct. The phenomenological orientations revealed by patients in Kerala also feature this apparent contradiction. They distinguish substance from spirit while also demonstrating awareness of mutual permutations of mind, body and other realms. However, Kerala phenomenology is not dualistic in the same way Western mind-body dualism is. As a continuum of states, it is not centered on a binary and mutually exclusive opposition between mind and body, but makes multiple fine distinctions between states consisting of greater and lesser degrees of physicality and tangibility.

Just as in Banaras, people in Kerala appreciate the material realm while idealizing the spirit. In Kerala, the intangible—analogous to Parry's term "spirit"—is highly valued and highly spoken of, yet in people's quotidian healing experiences they prefer a more pleasant aesthetic experience over one that is more abrasive. I would suggest, however, that this contradiction is found on the level of logic rather than on the level of experience. An esteem for the intangible self does not mean one is always able to live in this realm. It is something like a goal of experience, and it is one that is found in reflexive, literary, philosophical investigations.

Indian Philosophy and Phenomenology

Indian philosophical texts and popular mythology are saturated with discourses on the distinction between the self and the many "layers" of the person—including the self, consciousness, the mind, the subtle and gross bodies—and the nature of experience. By engaging philosophers such as Śankara, I am presenting an account of an Indian phenomenological orientation that is comparable to writings on the body and embodiment that invoke philosophers such as Descartes to characterize the Western mind-body dichotomy.[4] While Indian philosophy is to some degree an elite discourse, interviews with people in Kerala reveal that features of literate Indian philosophy and phenomenology also exist in popular discourse.

There are many positions and debates in Indian philosophy, and this section presents only a few key figures and ideas which are selected to reveal the genealogies and explicit exegeses of phenomenological terms used in contemporary illness discourses. Although Kerala is the focus here, most philosophical and phenomenological perspectives that are presented are part of a broader, Indian philosophical scene. Just how widely these perspectives are popularly consumed in other parts of India is beyond my ability to determine although evidence of a different popular phenomenological approach in an area of northern India will be presented later.

Defining and describing *ātman* is the concern of much Indian philosophical writing. Usually translated as "self" or "soul," *ātman* refers to a higher, ideal self that is described as totally immaterial and eternal and often wrongly, according to philosophers, identified with the mind or other personal attributes such as one's character, intelligence, name or personal history. *Ātman* is also a term that people I interviewed used to refer to something like an authentic self.

Identifying the nature of *ātman* was the primary concern of the philosopher Śankara. Born in the eighth century in what is now central Kerala, Śankara is known throughout India for his Advaita Vedānta philosophy, which aimed to demonstrate that the true self, *ātman*, is identical to *brahman* or god/the absolute. Śankara makes a considerable effort in his analyses to reveal phenomena that are wrongly attributed to *ātman* and must be recognized as such to realize this true self. Thinking that one's self is the body or that one perceives reality though the senses is erroneous according to Śankara. Even less tangible parts of the person, such as the mind or what we think of as one's personality, are not part of one's true identity, one's *ātman*. One perceives in Śankara a scale of decreasing tangibility as one goes from what in his estimation are false attributes to what is true and valued: from body to senses to mind to intellect to the completely intangible, nonmaterial *ātman*.

Early on in his treatise, *Upadeśa Sāhasrī*, Śankara emphasizes the Self's (i.e., *ātman*) separateness from the body:

> The Self, if in contact with the body, would be existing for the benefit of another and be non-eternal . . . . Moreover, the Self, supposed by other philosophers to be conjoined with the body must have an existence for the sake of another. (Śankaracharya 1973: 37)

In this passage, Śankara distinguishes himself from certain other philosophers including those he calls the "materialists," supporters of the Cārvāka school of skepticism, which advocates that reality consists only of what is perceived by the senses and that the self/soul exists only in the body.

In another section of *Upadeśa Sāhasrī*, Śankara narrates in the voice of *ātman*, and describes the nature of this self:

> Ever free, ever pure, changeless, immovable, immortal, imperishable and *bodiless* I have no knowledge or ignorance in Me who am of the nature of the Light of *Pure Consciousness only*. (Śankaracharya 1973: 121) [Emphasis added.]

This passage may help explain why in the following excerpts from interviews, people suffering illness appear concerned about their *bōdham* or "consciousness," which in its purest form is associated with *ātman* according to Śankara.

Śankara also distinguishes between mind (*manas*), intellect, memory and knowledge, all of which would be contained within the mind in Western epistemologies. He observes, for example, that "[t]he peculiar characteristic of the mind is reflection and that of the intellect is determination" (164). This distinction is seen in the various terms used by informants (such as *bōdham*, *buddhi* and *ōrmma*) that translate as "consciousness" or "intellect" yet are treated as distinct from "mind" (*manas*).

Śankara and his phenomenological views are known throughout Kerala and India. The popular religious leader Sai Baba, whose photo can be seen in homes and businesses in Kerala and other parts of India, promotes Śankara's philosophy that the true self is identical with the divine while other contemporary thinkers such as Vivekananda and Aurobindo have continued to develop his Advaita Vedānta philosophy.

Similar distinctions between the self, consciousness and the body are raised in a range of other works from fourth-century writings of Nyāya philosophy, which informs the methods and epistemologies of ayurvedic medicine, to the writings of the twentieth-century thinker, Sri Aurobindo.[5] This division or continuum of experiential instruments—body, mind, consciousness and *ātman*—can also be discerned in the contemporary narratives of people suffering possession and illness.

The distinctions between the material and tangible highlighted in these works could also be described using the distinction between gross (*sthūla*) and subtle (*sūkshma*) found in Indian philosophy and popular Hinduism. Substances are evaluated on a scale that ranges from the more gross to the more subtle (Marriott 1976) in which the subtle is more highly valued. Tantric Hinduism features a three level distinction between gross (*sthūla*), subtle (*sūkshma*) and supreme/transcendent (*parā*) (Brooks 1992) that may more closely resemble the phenomenological continuum I describe where the body is gross, *bōdham*/consciousness is subtle and *ātman* is transcendent.

The following comments by patients in Kerala depict an orientation to experience that resembles the phenomenology outlined in these textual, philosophical sources. In particular, Sanskritic terminology used in philosophical texts, such as *ātman*, *bōdham* and *manas*, is employed in contemporary discourse in Kerala along with a variety of idioms that translate roughly as "consciousness," suggesting a finely parsed awareness of states related to this realm of experience.

Bōdham, Manas and the Experience of Distress in Kerala

Intrigued by research on embodiment and its challenges to mind-body dualism, I hoped to find in India unique constellations of somatic idioms, forms of expression that offered an alternative to the modern, cosmopolitan, Western tendency to express distress in psychological idioms, but I was frustrated by my informants' propensity to talk about their problems in mentalistic and non-tangible terms. Although I modified my questions and advised my research assistants, who had some training in psychology, to veer away from questions that I thought might contain assumptions of mind-body dualism, I could not get informants to stop talking about their *manas* (mind) and their *bōdham* (consciousness). Finally, I conceded that something must be wrong with my theoretical orientations and the academic assumptions about the embodied Other on which they were based. Certainly some patients used embodied idioms or expressed their distress somatically, and it was sometimes apparent that informants' ways of speaking about their experience were conditioned by their embodied state. However, not one of the 38 patients for whom I have verbatim transcripts of interviews described their problems predominantly in somatic idioms or without referring to concerns about "consciousness," *ātman*, the mind or other non-tangible modes of experience. In fact, the elaborate nature of the mental and "consciousness"-oriented, perhaps metamental, terms patients used to describe their experience was striking to one accustomed to the vocabulary of Western mind-body dualism.

Treating Problems of the Mind

Several patients we interviewed described the explicitly mental nature of their suffering and how this related to the treatment they pursued. Two people we spoke with who were being treated at allopathic psychiatric hospitals explained that they sought help from a psychiatric hospital rather than from magic or sorcery because their particular problem came from "thinking." A 30-year-old male Muslim inpatient I call Hamid met with my assistant Kavitha and me at a private psychiatric hospital in Trivandrum. Hamid had been working, like many Malayalis, as a laborer in the United Arab Emirates before he returned home to seek relief for his problems, which included outbursts of anger, hallucinations and paranoia about his food being poisoned. His brother, who was present at our interview, explained that they first tried consulting ritual specialists, but then sought treatment at an allopathic psychiatric facility because of the mental nature of the problem:

> Brother of Hamid: After we came here [after his brother returned to Kerala], we took him to two or three places for *māntrika chikitsa* [black magic treatment].

> Kavitha: Where? In Beemapalli?

> Brother: No, near Beemapalli there is a place where we did *māntrika chikitsa.*

Kavitha: What all did they do?

Brother: They tied a thread and did their ritual. They did the rite in the Quran. Still he didn't get relief. So we saw another person who told us about the illness. He said the treatment for this can only be done in a hospital, and he can't do any *māntrika* [magic] for this. This occurred through thoughts [*chintāgathi*]. This began by thinking [*chintichchu untāyatānu*].

Jayasree is a retired school teacher who was in inpatient care at an allopathic psychiatric hospital for problems that included bouts of fear, sleeplessness, auditory hallucinations and a suicide attempt. In our conversation with Jayasree and her daughter, who are Hindu, her daughter explained why they were seeking treatment at a hospital rather than through *mantravādam* (magic/countersorcery):

Kavitha: Do you have some belief in that [referring to the possibility of involving magic or worship] relating to this problem?

Daughter of Jayasree: Not for this problem. This is because of *manas* [the mind].

Here and in other excerpts that follow, patients or their caretakers use the term *manas*, a Sanskrit-derived Malayalam word for mind that is also used in Indian philosophical texts. Although "mind" is the commonplace, dictionary translation of *manas*, this term refers to a realm of attributes that are not quite the same as those contained in the English "mind." In philosophical treatises, including the texts by Śankara discussed earlier and writings from the Vaiśeṣika school of thought, *manas* is distinct from *buddhi*, which is rendered as "intellect." Cognition and thinking are capacities of *manas*, but intellect and consciousness are not. *Manas* is a tool and more tangible, thereby further from the transcendent, disembodied *ātman* (the self) than the less tangible *bōdham* and *buddhi*. One might say that features or capacities that are encompassed in the English term "mind" are parsed into *manas, buddhi* and *bōdham* in India.

Occasionally, the distinction between mind and body is rendered in English terminology inserted into Malayalam narratives. In his first attempt to describe his troubles, Mohan, a 20-year-old male inpatient at an allopathic psychiatric hospital described his problem using the English term "mental" and explaining that his problems relate to thinking:

I have a "mental" [i.e., a mental problem]. I will think something. When asking someone something, I will feel different things in my mind. [. . .]

When I think like that, sometimes the anger inside me rises up to my mind. It will come up again. When I become like that I feel that I want to attack someone. Like that the thoughts will not stop.

Mohan also speaks about emotion, about his anger and his urge to attack someone. The description of anger rising to the mind reveals a connection between thought and emotion, but thoughts are Mohan's ultimate concern ("the thoughts will not stop"). At points throughout this interview, Mohan also expressed concern about his *ātman*. He felt that someone had taken his *ātman* and that it had merged with the *ātman* of another person: "There was a boy named R. R, I had a feeling that his *ātman* and my *ātman* have become one." This interview occurred early in the course of fieldwork, and Biju and I were still trying hard to elicit the somatic expressions, which were not appearing and we assumed were just hidden in the people we were speaking to. Mohan explicitly discounted our attempts to uncover somatic aspects of his problems:

Biju: Something else, do you have any other "strange physical feelings?" In your body, some kind of "strange feelings?"

Mohan: Nothing like that.

Murphy: "Okay, okay." [my indication to Biju that we ought to drop this line of questioning]

Mohan: No, this is only a "mental" illness. Other than that there is no illness.

Bōdham and Other Idioms of Consciousness

Mustapha, a 44-year-old Muslim fisherman who was seeking relief for his problems at Beemapalli mosque, was suffering an illness "in the head" according to his brother. This brother also related the onset of the problem to a loss of *bōdham*:

Kavitha: What all was he showing [i.e., what were his symptoms] when you took him to [name of mental hospital]?

Mustapha's Brother: I can't say exactly what he was showing when he became ill in the head. He will say things in reverse. He was brought back unconscious [*bōdhamillāte*].

A 32-year-old Hindu manual laborer was staying with his son, Satish, who was incarcerated in a cell (for uncontrollable or violent persons) while he sought relief for his suffering at Beemapalli mosque. Satish was around 18 years old and training to be a welder when his problem started. His father explained to me that a loss of *bōdham* was the defining characteristic of his son's problem:

Murphy: What all are the boy's problems?

Father: The problem is that one day when he was returning home after going to the road [where stores and services are found in the neighborhood] he had a feeling that hundreds of people were chasing him. He came and fell unconscious [*bōdham kettu*] at the doorstep. That's all there is to the illness. There is nothing other than that.

Lakshmi, the Hindu woman introduced in Chapter 3 who had been attending Chottanikkara temple to seek the goddess' help with her problems described her experience of possession in terms of several interior and exterior levels of *bōdham*:

Biju: Do you have consciousness [*bōdham*] during possession [*tullāl*]? Consciousness [*bōdham*]?

Lakshmi: No.

Biju: Do you have consciousness inside [*ullil bōdham kānumō*]?

Lakshmi: Inside the inside, there will be consciousness [*ullinte ullil bōdham kānum*]. The reason is . . . but there is no outside. There is a feeling that something is inside.

Biju: No consciousness [*bōdham*] on the outside, right?

Lakshmi: No consciousness [*bōdhamilla*].

Lakshmi is referring to a level of interiority where there is awareness of what is occurring during possession although her normal state of *bōdham* is not active or is not perceiving what is going on around and within her.

A woman who was receiving outpatient psychiatric treatment, in her first attempt to describe her problem, resorts to the idiom *bōdham*, but also uses a term, *ōrmma*, which has a meaning similar to "consciousness" but can also refer to "memory:" "I lost memory/consciousness [*Ōrmmayillāteyāyi*]. Yesterday night, I became unconscious [*bōdhamillāteyāyi*]."

An unemployed Hindu woman whose husband works as a manual laborer for the railways and who was a psychiatric inpatient at Trivandrum Medical

College Hospital, explained the primary characteristics of her illness using *ōrmma*:

> Like this I was unconsciously [*ōrmmayillāte*] saying things. I called my mother bad names. I was unconscious [*ōrmmayilla*]. I could not eat anything.

In this passage, it is difficult to ascertain whether it is better to render *ōrmma* as "memory" or "consciousness," two of its English glosses. The following incident involving an elderly patient, Kuttappan, at the Government Ayurveda Mental Hospital helps clarify some of the meanings of this idiom:

> Wife of Kuttappan: We can't sleep here. Yesterday, his son was here with him. He beat him [the son] with a flashlight.
>
> Benny: His son?
>
> Wife of Kuttapan: Yes. There was a cut here, and a tooth was hit and loosened.
>
> Kuttappan: I don't remember [*ōrmmayilla*] that.
>
> Benny: He did it unconsciously [*ōrmmayillāte*].
>
> Wife of Kuttapan: Unconsciously [*ōrmmayillāte*], he did it. So they chained him. I told him to bring tea in the morning. His son had not had tea. It was to soothe him. So ask your son. Father did that unconsciously. So let him call his son and ask him whether he had tea. Then he started crying. At that time he was not in his conscious mind [more literally, he was of little intellect—*buddhikku lēsham*].

Kuttappan's wife referred to her husband as lacking *buddhi*, which is a term used in Nyāya, Vaiśesika and other philosophies to refer to the intellect, a capacity that is not the same as *manas* (mind) or the body. *Buddhi* is less tangible, more subtle and more highly valued than mind and body. In this excerpt, *ōrmma* appears to be a type of consciousness or awareness that can be linked to past events, but the following exchange with a Christian woman who was at Vettucaud church appealing for relief for her daughter, Teresa—a fish vendor who had started swearing, acting violently and causing trouble for her family—shows that the association between *ōrmma* and memory is not automatic:

> Kavitha: When she is having this problem, are there any memory [*ōrmma*] problems?
>
> Mother of Teresa: Sometimes she will be unconscious [*ōrmmayillāte kitakkum*]. Then we will warm her up by giving her something hot to drink and all.

Kavitha: No, *ōrmma*. Does she have *ōrmma* for past events and all?

Mother of Teresa: There is no problem like that.

Ōrmma is thus evocative of a type of consciousness that is usually, but not always, related to the past.

The relative of Mahmud, a young Muslim man who was an inpatient at the Government Ayurveda Mental Hospital (GAMH), brought up another expression that one of my assistants felt was also best rendered as (loss of) "consciousness:"

> He lost consciousness [*talakku oru marichchal*—lit.: a turning in his head] is what he is saying. He lost consciousness [*talakku oru marichchal*]. After that, he won't talk. He speaks only with his arms and legs.

Another patient at the GAMH, a young Hindu man, brought up yet another term that my assistants and I thought best translated as "unconscious." Sivan had angry, sometimes violent, outbursts, and his family had taken him to an allopathic psychiatric hospital before coming to the GAMH. Both types of facilities are seen as places that can treat problems involving the mind and "consciousness." In attempting to explain the origin of his problems, Sivan recalled:

> Sivan: They [friends who had threatened him] made me sick.
>
> Benny: Who did this, and how did they make you sick?
>
> Sivan: They made me unconscious [*mayakki*].
>
> Benny: Made you unconscious [*mayakkiyō*]?
>
> Sivan: Made me unconscious and scolded me [*Mayakkittu parihasichchittu*].

Maya/mayakkuka can also refer to intoxication, confusion, coma, enchantment and dimness (Madhavanpillai 1976). One could interpret, given these additional meanings, that *maya* is a more embodied form of (un)consciousness, states like intoxication or coma requiring a relationship to the body to be experienced. Or perhaps, consciousness being absent, one has dropped down to the level of the body or the tangible, like Mahmud above who "speaks only with his arms and legs" after losing consciousness.

A 35-year-old Hindu man, Santhosh, who was employed part-time at a photo studio was an inpatient at the state-run, allopathic Mental Health

Centre in Trivandrum when we met him. His first attempt to describe his problem invokes another idiom that, again lacking terminology for such finely parsed states of consciousness in English, we had to render as "consciousness":

> Biju: What are the symptoms [*lakshananngal*—lit., characteristics] of your illness?

> Santhosh: Symptoms of illness? When I sleep I will fall into a deep sleep without any consciousness [*ariyān vayāte uranngum*—or "I will sleep without being able to know"].

These patient accounts reveal an attention to distinctions of "consciousness" that are reminiscent of the concerns of Indian philosophers. Lakshmi's reference to consciousness remaining "inside the inside" during possession, for example, resembles Śankara's effort to characterize *ātman* as the "witness" of all that occurs in the mind and consciousness. For people suffering "mental" distress in Kerala, these various types of "consciousness" represent a predominant area of concern related to their suffering, a place of rupture in their selfhood or state of being that is expressed as an illness. These modes of "consciousness" constitute a realm that is less tangible than body or the mind (*manas*), and represent an orientation to experience that cannot be characterized in terms of (Western) mind-body dualism.

Relations Between Tangible and Intangible Modes of Experience

People in Kerala *do* express suffering through the body in addition to their mental and consciousness-based modes of expression. However, people suffering distress who attend to their bodies appear more concerned about their states of *manas* (mind) and *bōdham* (consciousness).

A Hindu woman, Santhi, who was receiving inpatient treatment at the Trivandrum Medical College expresses her difficulties through a combination of somatic and disembodied idioms. Santhi was having financial difficulties at home, she was worried about her husband's drinking, and she complained that her mother-in-law mistreats her. "Thinking [*vichārichchā*] about all this," Santhi explained, "I have mental troubles [*manassinu vishamam*]." But, she later added, her problem also appears in bodily and aesthetic forms:

> When I try to sleep in the daytime, sometimes I feel like my legs are shaking, like my legs are moving and my head is heavy. And when my head is heavy, I think I will lose my normal state/mind [*samanila tetti pōkum*].

Santhi's problem manifests itself in the body, but this description culminates in her concern about losing her state of mind. Here heaviness affects the mind, perhaps relating to the sense that the mind is somewhat material, or at least more tangible than *bōdham* and other types of consciousness. Returning to the somatic aspects of her suffering, Santhi explained:

Santhi: Now when my body becomes *chenattu kayaru* [numb/limp/stiff] and when I am tired.

Kavitha: What is "*chenattu kayaru*"?

Santhi: All this hair will stand up straight. It will go away after a while.

Kavitha: Is this the only thing you feel, or is there anything else?

Santhi: Sometimes I will have stomach pain, burning in the chest. Sometimes burning in the stomach, then headache. Everything is there.

Santhi then responds to Kavitha's prompt to talk about mental and bodily states, but she emphasizes that her fear—which in this exchange seems to be the most crucial concern about her illness—relates to her mental state:

Kavitha: You said that this will happen [that you will be possessed]. When that happens, how do you feel in your body? And in your mind, how do you feel?

Santhi: In my mind, I will be afraid.

Kavitha: Will be afraid. Other than that?

Santhi: Nothing other than that.

Kavitha: Nothing more than that.

Santhi: I am afraid. I feel that I will lose my normal mind [*samanila tetti pōkum*].

The mother of Sreedevi, the woman introduced in Chapter 3 who was seeking ayurvedic psychiatric treatment and was worried about whether she could get married, described Sreedevi's difficulties in terms of bodily, behavioral and emotional idioms:

Biju: What is the problem for which you are seeking treatment?

Sreedevi's Mother: She is not eating, and she has started crying. And when sleeping, she'll suddenly wake up complaining of stomach pain. She shows *bahalam* [agitation/boisterousness].

But then Sreedevi's mother explains:

Because this is a mental problem [*manassikamāyittulla vishamam*], we have been coming here.

All these excerpts reveal features of culturally defined phenomenological experience. The phenomenological orientation engaged by patients in Kerala is marked by several modes of experience that range from the more material to the more intangible, subtle and rarefied: that is, from the body to *manas* (mind) to *bōdham* (consciousness) to *ātman*. The other idioms of "consciousness" offered by informants, such as *ōrmma* and *buddhi*, lie between *manas* and *ātman* on this continuum of modes of experience. The people we spoke with do not explicitly say that these modes of experience lie on a continuum of increasing intangibility, but they use these terms in a way that is consistent with the philosophies described earlier, which outline a continuum of body-mind-consciousness-*ātman*. Patients' concerns for their more subtle states of experience were also highlighted in the analysis of the preceding interviews. In addition, it is noteworthy that in the first set of excerpts, which focused on explanations for seeking treatment, interviewees referred to the terms *manas* (mind) and problems of thinking to explain why they pursued psychiatric therapy, allopathic or ayurvedic. In later excerpts, when patients were recounting their more personal, proximate experiences of illness, terminology focused more on idioms of consciousness (*bōdham, ōrmma*) or losing consciousness (*mayakkuka*). This indicates that the various styles of consciousness are likely more experience-near, more personally valued modes of experience while *manas*, in addition to being more mechanical and tangible, appears more depersonalized and pragmatic.

Unlike many other ethnographic examples in anthropological studies of the body, some of which are discussed at the outset of this chapter, people suffering affliction and illness in Kerala do distinguish mind from body and locate experience in emphatically disembodied and highly valued, non-tangible realms. Yet, mind and body are not diametrically opposed in Kerala as they are in Western mind-body dualism. They are simply different, and in fact mind—*manas*—is more embodied, more gross and material, and thus closer to the body than *bōdham* and *ātman*. Mind and body are only parts, and not even the focal parts, of an experiential orientation that, if anything, is most concerned about *bōdham, ōrmma* and other states of consciousness.

The preceding examples present similar orientations in people from various class, gender and religious backgrounds, but further investigation may reveal variations along these lines. Class, caste, gender, religion and linguistic differences may well correspond to varied phenomenological sensibilities within Kerala and throughout India. In fact, the Indian philosophies described earlier are to some degree elite discourses, but what may make Kerala unique is that these elite philosophies and phenomenologies seem to be popularly consumed.

Kerala State Phenomenology?

Living in Kerala, one becomes accustomed to the variety of acronyms for high-profile programs developed by the state government—from the KSRTC (Kerala State Road Transportation Corporation) buses that ply the roads of every town in the state to the reliable but modest KTDC (Kerala Tourist Development Corporation) hotels to the KSFDC (Kerala State Film Development Corporation) whose festivals promote prestigious independent directors. Although the Government of Kerala extends its reach into many aspects of civic life, it would be odd to imagine a particular phenomenology, a way of experiencing the world, associated with this modern state, yet people's phenomenological orientations appear to be associated with processes of the modern state as well as other, earlier features of place. Key elements of contemporary phenomenological orientations can be found in the Malayalam language and the philosophical views of the person, both lay and literate, that go back hundreds of years, and there are contemporary social processes and state practices that have a role in how people in contemporary Kerala experience the world and, in particular, "mental" distress.

One assertion of this study is that phenomenological orientations vary by place and time, and social and historical practices have helped shape the phenomenological orientation that organizes and mediates experience among people I spoke to in Kerala. We may be seeing this process in action as people in Kerala engage with Western/biomedical idioms of distress, such as "tension" and "depression," which accompany the proliferation of biomedical psychiatric services and discourses.

The expressions of distress exhibited by patients in Kerala differ from those Langford (1998) observed at an ayurvedic psychotherapy practice in north India. According to Langford, many patients of ayurvedic therapist Dr. Singh present somatic symptoms (e.g., weakness, stomach pain, constipation) which the doctor diagnoses as a problem with *vata* (one of the *dosas*, the underlying essences of the body) (89–90). One patient Langford observed was described as unusual in that he complained of "extreme depression" (90). Paraphrasing the view of an ayurvedic therapist regarding this case, Langford explained: "In India . . . there is not much awareness about psychological problems. Usually people with psychological disorders come to the outpatient department complaining of physical ailments and are diagnosed by Dr. Singh with depression and/or anxiety" (91). By contrast, many of the people I interviewed characterized their psychological problems primarily in terms of what could be called "psychological" states—that is, states of *manas, bōdham* and *ātman*—rather than physical ailments.

It is tempting to consider that people in Kerala may de-emphasize the body and prioritize the more intangible parts of the person because of the influence of Western, allopathic medicine. As mentioned earlier, allopathy is far more prolific in Kerala than in other states of India.[6] However, there is no simple hegemony of biomedicine in Kerala. The state has as many ayurvedic facilities as it has allopathic facilities, but there are more allopathic beds and doctors (State Planning Board, cited in Mani 1998). There are also more ayurvedic doctors who specialize in *manasika rōgam* (mental illness) compared to other regions of India (Kakar 1982, Bhattacharyya 1986). Thus it would be questionable to argue that people in Kerala are simply adopting allopathic perspectives in "psychologizing" forms of distress that are exhibited somatically in other parts of India. In addition, elements of the phenomenological orientations engaged by people in Kerala predate the arrival of biomedicine in South Asia, and as demonstrated by patient accounts, differ from Western mind-body phenomenology. In addition, the phenomenological perspectives presented here come not only from informants undergoing allopathic psychiatric therapy but also from persons who were using ayurvedic therapy and religious healing, although allopathic psychological and psychiatric discourse is broadly disseminated through television, film and the print media.

On the other hand, the phenomenological orientations people engage with in Kerala are not static, and it is possible that the supremacy of the intangible parts of the person is reinforced by the privileging of mind over body in Western biomedical discourses, which are well known and, in some contexts, prestigious in Kerala. Although the two phenomenologies diverge, the Western biomedical orientation being more dualistic and the orientation among patients in Kerala representing more of a finely graded continuum, the valuing of mind over body resembles the prioritizing of the intangible over the tangible.

It is also possible that the phenomenological orientation people engage with in Kerala relates to the state's achievement of near total literacy. While the current literacy rate can certainly be attributed to grassroots and government literacy programs that have been implemented in the last few decades, literacy has historically been a distinguishing feature of Kerala/Malayali society. Gough (1968) cites examples of the local consumption of elite Sanskritic sources and literacy in Malayalam from the ninth, sixteenth and other centuries. What we may be seeing in Kerala is the popular consumption of what, in other parts of India, would be elite phenomenological discourses. The philosophical views I have presented represent high, literate culture in various parts of India, but in Kerala they are also popularly engaged to a significant degree. Today in Kerala, literacy enables the consumption of biomedical psychiatric and medical discourse through popular media, such as psychological advice columns in magazines such as *Mangalam* and *Manorama* and television shows that feature biomedical experts. Again the picture is complex: while biomedical views receive more coverage, ayurvedic doctors and other healers also appear in the popular media and have a role in shaping popular illness discourses. Popular magazines also occasionally feature columnists and essayists who present concepts that stem from Indian philosophy in writing about the self and "psychological" topics (topics related to understanding the self and the emotions, although not necessarily engaging Western psychological discourse).

Mind-body dualism has added another set of idioms for articulating distress that many in Kerala have mixed in to their local phenomenological orientation. It is ironic that, vis-a-vis contemporary academic studies of the body, mind-body dualism has provided a more embodied phenomenological language to describe and perhaps experience states of distress. I suggest that English metaphors of "psychological" distress that have been adopted in Kerala belie a greater attention to embodied experience than metaphors of distress that are used in Malayalam.

Malayalam idioms (usually Sanskritic words borrowed into Malayalam) indicating various non-bodily states exist in Kerala discourse alongside a variety of English language terms for distress. For example, in Chapter 3 we saw both Mary and Hanifa describe their problems using the word "tension." Meanwhile, Rajan, who had sought treatment at Chottanikkara temple, spoke of "depression" in describing the experience of possession:

Biju: Can you talk about how it "feels" when we get "possessed?"

Rajan: I will tell you. We know suddenly when someone scares us from behind we get frightened, right? Then what "depression" we would feel. That is, that "depression" is the "first" thing we will feel.

The English idioms of distress "tension," "depression" and "stress" are metaphors that are kinetic or convey a sense of physical torsion—they suggest a feeling of pressure or weight on the body in order to represent problems attributed to the mind or emotion. Malayalam and Sanskritic terms for distress do not evoke these senses. Malayalam idioms used by people I spoke to in Kerala who were suffering distress include: *vishamam*, which best translates as "sadness," *kashtanngal*, which means "troubles," and *dukham*, which is best rendered as "grief." A greater knowledge of Malayalam etymology and a thorough analysis of these words in their use in everyday discourse would be necessary, however, to complete this comparison more accurately. In addition, while privileging mind over body is similar to valuing the intangible over the tangible, the phenomenology in Kerala locates both mind and body on the lower, more material and tangible end of the body-mind-*bōdham-ātman* continuum. Yet both phenomenologies do have in common a denigration of the body.

Chapter 5 continues the focus on phenomenological features of health and healing, but examines the more tangible realms of the person through an analysis of the aesthetic experience of undergoing therapy. Although patients are most concerned about the intangible parts of the person, given the choice between several therapeutic options, they prefer a process of healing that more pleasantly, or less abrasively, engages the tangible aspects of experience. *Ātman* does not require austerities and physical suffering to be realized, at least not in the realm of healing. Meanwhile, it should be recalled that the mind/*manas* is partially tangible, and a viscerally agreeable healing experience, ideally a "cooling" experience, is for many a more appealing way to seek relief from mental distress.

Notes

1. On locating the Other in time see Fabian (1983) and Augé (1999 [1994]).
2. See Bordo (1993) and Gilbert (1997) on women's bodies, Fishburn's (1997) study of the African-American body in literary narratives and Kleinman (1986) and Scheper-Hughes (1992) on working class bodies.
3. Kleinman explained that so-called "mental" problems are somatically expressed throughout most of the world:

    > The research literature indicates that depression and most other mental illnesses, especially in non-Western societies and among rural, ethnic and lower-class groups in the West, are associated preponderantly with physical complaints. (1986:52)

    Kleinman's claim was supported by much research in cross-cultural psychiatry. A WHO-funded study found that a majority of psychiatric patients at primary health care facilities in "developing country" sites (India, Colombia, Sudan and the Philippines) presented with physical complaints (Climent et al. 1980,

158 ~ CHAPTER 4

Harding et al. 1980). However, more recent psychiatric research claims that somatization is not the more common expression of distress in "developing countries"
(Piccinelli and Simon 1997).

The "developed/developing" dichotomy used by cross-cultural psychiatrists
in their research on somatization mirrors the "Western/non-Western" dichotomy used by anthropologists in their studies of the body. Psychiatric researchers
use socioeconomic categories whereas anthropologists use cultural difference to
divide the world into the somatic and the mental.

4. Such as Scheper-Hughes and Lock (1987), Csordas (1994) and Strathern (1996:
   41–62).
5. Radhakrishnan and Moore, eds. (1957: 356–385, 602–603).
6. With only 4% of India's population, Kerala had 30% of the allopathic mental
   hospitals in India in 1991 (Franke and Chasin 1994:v, citing *India Abroad*, Dec.
   13, 1991, p. 32). Also, Bhattacharyya's research in Bengal (1986) and Nunley's
   work in Uttar Pradesh (1996) reveal that biomedical psychiatric services in those
   regions are not as prevalent as they are in Kerala.

5

꧁

COOLING MUDPACKS: THE AESTHETIC
QUALITY OF THERAPY

I first became aware of the importance of attending to the aesthetic quality of the process of therapy one afternoon while I was at the Government Ayurveda Mental Hospital observing the administrations of inpatient psychiatric procedures. One patient who was undergoing *talapodichil*—the procedure described in Chapter 2 wherein nurses apply a medicated "mudpack" to the patient's head and cover it with a banana leaf—joked about how silly his banana leaf "hat" looked but also explained that the treatment provided a pleasant, cooling effect. Meanwhile, patients who were receiving *nasya* laughed because of the tickling they experienced as medicines were poured into their noses and their heads were massaged. I thought how strikingly this differed from the atmosphere I had observed around inpatient allopathic psychiatric procedures. Electroconvulsive therapy, for example, was always a somewhat traumatic procedure. Far from being "cooling," a common description for positive aesthetic experiences in Kerala, electroconvulsive therapy was considered unpleasant or painful, and humor was inappropriate.

I further examined patient appraisals of their aesthetic experiences in different therapies, and learned that adverse effects of medications and electroconvulsive therapy have led some to discontinue allopathic psychiatric therapy and pursue other types of treatment. In addition to discovering that patients prefer a more pleasant process of therapy during psychiatric treatment, I realized that a pleasant, aesthetically engaging process could also in itself serve as a kind of "cure" or resolution for some patients' problems. After speaking with the family of a woman who had had behavioral problems for years and who was seeking relief simply by praying at Vettucaud church, I realized that several people we met had sought relief for their problems for several years—often including several stays at mental hospitals—and had been living for an extended period at a mosque, temple or church. Perhaps these individuals had given up on treatment to a certain degree and found a resolution, a paradoxically nonteleological "solution" to their problems by remaining in a pleasant environment, a scenic setting with music, chanting, incense, flowers and a chance to engage one's spirituality. Some of these people, who have been struggling with mental problems for years and could be considered incurable in psychiatric terms, had found a resolution to their problems that was distinct from the ideal of cure. They found a way to cope with an intractable illness by living with their problems in the aesthetically engaging setting of a mosque, temple or church, essentially living in a pleasant process of therapy.

This attention to the process of healing further problematizes the concepts of cure and healing. The cultural contingency of the idea of cure and the goals of treatment are highlighted by patients' and their caretakers' descriptions of the variety of states that are attained through therapy, such as improvement, living in the process of therapy and achieving a better-than-normal state. This analysis suggests that an overemphasis on curing in allopathic psychiatry may obscure attention to the aesthetic quality of undergoing a therapy.

Considering the pleasantness of the process of treatment, which refers not just to pleasant sensations but to the relative degrees of pleasantness and abrasiveness in undergoing treatment, reworks our understandings of healing in two ways that are significant for researchers and practitioners who work on mental health. First, and simply, one ought to consider how pleasant or painful it is to undergo therapy. Patients appreciate a pleasant or less violent method of therapy, and the pleasantness of the therapeutic process affects patients' choice of therapy and their decision to continue treatment. Second, the fact that some people who are suffering distress in Kerala have found a way to manage their problems by continuing to live with an intractable illness in a pleasant environment and others feel they have achieved a state that is somehow better or higher than their normal, healthy state, suggests that researchers should broaden their understanding of what is accomplished in treatment. Practitioners should meanwhile be aware of how the ideals of curing might affect treatment and consider a more diverse realm of therapeutic dispensations, including less teleological orientations, in coping with mental suffering.

My interest in the connection between the process and resolution of healing was also inspired by my realization that the term "cure" has no direct translation in the Malayalam language. "Cure" refers to the eradication of a problem or a return to a state of health—often defined simply as a lack of illness—that existed prior to the development of a pathology. People in Kerala, however, talk of bringing "change" (*māruka/māttam*), finding "improvement" (*bhēdam*) or even reaching a state of "prosperity" (*abhivriddhi*) to invoke a few Malayalam expressions for what is accomplished through healing. Some of these expressions are more modest and incremental while others are more exalted than the ideal of curing.

"Pleasant" is used here to describe a variety of experiences in undergoing treatment that are at times pleasant and at least non-abrasive. The everyday meanings of this word are inadequate to cover the range of issues discussed here, but rather than invent a term to describe these aesthetic features, I will define the various meanings I am attributing to the word "pleasant." Often "pleasant" appropriately describes a person's positive sensorial reaction to a method of treatment. For example, "cooling" (*tanuppu, kulirmma*) is a commonly heard local idiom for expressing the positively-valued aesthetic experience some people reported in undergoing therapy in Kerala.

"Pleasant" can, however, be too positive a term to describe therapies that are simply *less* abrasive to undergo. Ayurveda, for example, can be uncomfortable, irritating or demanding, requiring one to undergo an austere vegetarian diet, digest a large quantity of *ghee* (clarified butter) or take medicine to induce vomiting. But there remains a difference between the adverse aspects of ayurvedic and allopathic treatments. While ayurvedic treatment could be characterized as at times uncomfortable or demanding, according to patients' reports of their experiences in therapy, allopathic therapies can at times be painful, disconcerting or, occasionally, traumatic. Another way to characterize the difference is that both ayurvedic and allopathic treatments involve therapies that are unpleasant to undergo, but only ayurveda features treatments that patients describe as creating pleasant aesthetic effects. These are not necessarily essential, eternal characteristics of these therapies. As will be discussed later, there is evidence that in the past ayurveda used more invasive, violent therapies and allopathy was more focused than it is now on care and giving relief.

There are also occasions where "pleasant" is too mundane to describe the transformative experience, the bringing-to-a-higher-level, some people say they experience in healing. The demanding nature of ayurveda is sometimes described as part of the process of cultivating self-discipline, or a development of the self that some say occurs in therapy. This is similar to a spiritual benefit reported by patrons of religious healing in Kerala. Healing in these cases is not just "pleasant" in the visceral or aesthetic sense, but somewhat exalted, a raising of the self or spirit to a higher level, not just a healing in the sense of removing a problem or returning to normalcy, but a transformation to a more auspicious state.

Also implicated in this examination of process and cure is what could be seen as differing orientations toward time in therapy. Allopathic treatment in the situations described in this section can be seen as more teleological, gazing ahead toward the desired end result and less concerned about the quality of the process of undergoing treatment. Ayurveda meanwhile can be seen as attending more intently to the passage of time in therapy, to the nature of the experience of undergoing treatment. Although remission of symptoms and a return to a state of health, or an enhanced state of health, is usually the ideal goal in ayurvedic therapy, the aesthetic quality of the process of treatment is emphasized while working toward this goal. In the religious therapies, consideration of the quality of the process of therapy is also present, though the process can be subsumed in a broader effort to achieve a spiritual transformation. There are also contexts where healing in religious therapies lacks a clear goal or attention to the passage of time. For example, while some say prayer helps to attain relief, the actual moment of prayer itself *is* relief from suffering for some individuals.

I do not claim to present a neat fit between the phenomenological orientation described in the previous chapter and the attention to "pleasantness." The concern over pleasant or cooling experiences and their positive effects on the mind attest to the partial tangibility of the mind in relation to other parts of the person. Essentially, this chapter engages with the partially material realm of truly "mental" (in the sense of *manas,* the partly tangible mental faculty of Indian phenomenology) healing, and reinforces the observation that Kerala phenomenology is not mind-body dualism. The issues in this chapter engage with effects on *manas*/mind and something like the "sense organs" (though patients do not use this ayurvedic category that refers to the somewhat material instruments that are responsible for sensory engagement), the partially tangible, partially intangible area that lies between the tangible body and the disembodied *ātman* on the phenomenological continuum engaged by patients in Kerala. Patients speak of cooling the mind but not *bōdham* which is not discussed in terms of physical sensations. Though the greatest concern for several patients presented in the last chapter relates to *ātman*, this is an ideal part of the person that is difficult to engage, and in the realm of healing at least, one does not need to suffer physically in order to realize or embrace this authentic self. Given a choice between several roads to improve one's mental health or consciousness in Kerala's medically pluralistic setting, some more pleasant than others, people prefer the more pleasant option. This is not the case in all realms of experience though. In certain ritual contexts, such as the Sabarimala pilgrimage to a mountaintop temple, ideally undertaken by foot, and Taipooja rituals, physical austerities and suffering *are* part of realizing one's higher self.

The Aesthetics of Healing

Carol Laderman and Marina Roseman (1996) offered the insight that "if healing is to be effective or successful, the senses must be engaged" (4), but we also need to ask whether some therapies invoke more pleasant sensory reactions than others. Studies of the aesthetics of healing have neither compared different therapies nor examined the aesthetics of western biomedicine. This may be due to the fact that aesthetic studies of healing focus on therapies such as shamanistic healing that are more patently, more dramatically sensual. An awareness of the feel, smell and color of Nepalese shamanistic healing (Desjarlais 1992) and Chinese medicine (Farquhar 2002) is crucial for making sense of the healing process, but the aesthetic characteristics of these healing systems would take on an additional value if contrasted to the aesthetic experience of undergoing biomedical treatment. Biomedical practitioners do not explicitly try to create an aesthetic environment. Patients and healers do not light incense and sing at biomedical facilities, and the main aesthetic experiences are the effects of treatment or the sterile and putatively neutral environment of the clinic, which, ironically, has its own "feel." In addition, biomedical practitioners sometimes need to suppress the aesthetics of therapy through the use of *an*aesthetics. Thus, aesthetic experience appears to be something that one tries to avoid in allopathic practice, and perhaps the lack of an effort to create a positive aesthetic environment, the lack of an alternative aesthetic for the patient to focus on, or the inadvertent creation of an uninspiring hospital aesthetic (the flat, modern interior, and the vaguely antiseptic smell of the clinic), leads patients to focus more intently on the visceral effects of treatment.

The Concept of "Cure" and the Ends of Healing

Little attention has been devoted to the concept of curing in social analyses of health and illness. The term "cure" is applied in many medical contexts by anthropologists and others, and its allopathic assumptions are usually taken for granted as what one tries to do with an illness.[1]

Anthropologists who study chronic illness have occasionally reflected on the meaning of cure and the goals of therapy. Estroff (1981) in her ethnography of people suffering psychopathology while trying to cope with daily life in non-institutional, community settings in the U.S. addressed the meaning of "cure:" "I had expected that people in the treatment program would be cured or would get better. I did not know that the process and progress would be so slow, so painful, and so laden with failure and setbacks" (18). The situation of the people Estroff describes is reminiscent of individuals in Kerala who have chosen to live with intractable psychopathologies at a temple, mosque or church having essentially given up on attempting to overcome their illness. Additionally, Kleinman (1988a) proposed emphasizing care rather than cure among people with chronic illnesses, asserting that "chronic illness by definition cannot be cured, that indeed the quest for cure is a dangerous myth that serves patient and practitioner poorly" (229). Estroff and Kleinman did not elaborate on how the concept of cure is constructed, but their recognition of its significance to those seeking therapy foreshadows this chapter's concern with examining its cross-cultural implications.

Although he does not aim his critique at the ideology of cure specifically, Alter's (1999) work on the principle of health in ayurveda complements my scrutiny of the goals of healing as he points to a "remedial bias" in medical anthropology and contemporary medical practices (44). Alter claims that in ayurveda health is seen as ongoing improvement rather than a concern for restoring balance or removing illness. Analyses of healing in various cultural contexts, Alter suggests, have overemphasized remedial, oppositional and curative approaches to health. Like the ideology of curing, the "remedial bias" tends to isolate healing practices from approaches to health that engage in broader projects of improvement and transformation.

The concept of cure is problematized in several ways by the experience of patients in Kerala. First, patient experiences alert us to the importance of balancing caring and curing, of attending to the quality of the process of therapy while "fighting" an illness. Second, living in an aesthetically- and spiritually-engaging environment as a means of coping with a problem constitutes an alternative to the goal of eradication of an illness that is implied in seeking a cure. Finally, there are patients who felt they achieved a state that is better or more exalted than the remission of symptoms or return to a pre-illness state that is inherent in the concept of curing. That is, they claim they attained a state of well-being that is more vibrant, more robust than what they experienced before their illness. Recalling Alter's claims about the goals of ayurvedic therapy, we can say in this context that "health" is seen not simply as a lack of illness, or as a default or baseline state of being. As implied by the Malayalam term *sukham*, which translates equally well as "health," "well-being" and "happiness," "health" can be something that is constantly improved upon, a presence of well-being or vibrance which, ideally, can be continually enhanced.

The concept of cure and the degree of emphasis on this goal may explain what I saw as a lesser attention to the aesthetic quality of the process of therapy in allopathic psychiatry in Kerala. However, this analysis of the ideology of cure in biomedicine is somewhat incipient. There are issues that would require additional investigation to more fully evaluate the implications of the ideal of curing. For example, there is a difference between the ideals of biomedicine and its practice, and there exists a diversity of practices within biomedicine that can undermine any universal claims about this medical system.[2] I also want to emphasize that I am not suggesting biomedicine is at all times exclusively focused on curing, on the final results of therapy. As will be discussed below, some diseases are considered chronic or incurable, and some physicians work only on easing suffering. I suggest that it is the *degree* of emphasis on cure and how this ideal shapes practice that leads to a lesser attention to the pleasantness of the process of treatment. Furthermore, it is not simply the concept behind a single term, "cure," that requires investigation, but the practices and the variety of goals associated with the ideal of the removal of a pathogen and restoration of "health"—such as the use of invasive techniques, efforts to eradicate a pathogen and attempts to relieve symptoms—that merit scrutiny.

The biomedical and history of medicine literatures give us some, though limited, insight into the origins, the historical trajectories and the contemporary meaning of cure in biomedicine. Biomedical literature reveals little discussion of the meaning of cure, reflecting perhaps the underscrutinized, taken-for-granted nature of this ideal. "Cure" is not defined in *Black's Medical Dictionary*, or in most medical dictionaries and reference books I reviewed at a major medical school library. Also, no definition of cure is brought up in any psychiatric or general medical textbook I examined. One medical dictionary that did define "cure" did so as follows:

> 1. restoration of health of a person afflicted with a disease or other disorder. 2. the favorable outcome of the treatment of a disease or other disorder. 3. a course of therapy, a medication, a therapeutic measure, or another remedy used in treatment of a medical problem ... (*Mosby's Medical, Nursing & Allied Health Dictionary* 2002: 459).

The *Oxford English Dictionary*'s fifth definition for "cure", "[t]o heal (a disease or wound); *fig.* to remedy, rectify, remove (an evil of any kind)," contains the notion of *removing*, which I would argue is an assumption in contemporary allopathic practice that is not covered in the medical dictionary definition above. Also, the *Oxford English Dictionary* in its first entry for "cure" gives the definition "To take care of; to care for, regard", a now defunct usage[3] which nevertheless evokes the overlap between process and final disposition, or care and cure, I observed in Kerala.

This original meaning of "cure" is invoked by historians of biomedicine who claim that a division arose in the past between efforts to take *care* of the ill (make them feel better) and *cure* the patient (remove the disease entity). Kothari and Mehta warn against the tendency in "modern medicine" (allopathy/biomedicine) to utilize invasive procedures to remove any abnormality and other instances of what they see as violence in medical practice. They suggest that healers should focus on easing dis-ease (the pain in suffering) and thereby return medicine to the original meaning of "cure," which was "to take care:"

> The idea that the chief role of a medical system is to take care of the dis-eased gives the system only a palliative role. This is as it should be. Oliver Wendell Holmes has described his teacher, Dr. Jackson, as one who never talked of curing his patients "except in its true etymological sense of taking care of him." . . .

> Modern medicine is in need of humility; it must give back to "cure" its etymological meaning. It must recognize that with a concerned physician around, no disease, no death, is incurable. A drug to ease, a procedure to palliate, a word of cheer, the graceful stoicism to hold the dying patient's hand—all this and more falls within the curative competence of a compassionate clinician (1988: 197).

This proposal differs from the present status of palliative care in allopathic medicine. "Palliative" is defined as "a term applied to the treatment of incurable diseases, in which the aim is to mitigate the sufferings of the patient, not to effect a cure" (*Black's Medical Dictionary* 1992: 434), and palliative care focuses on terminally ill patients and hospice care (Doyle et al. 1998). Palliative medicine thus refers to attempts to relieve suffering after the possibility of cure has passed—although Chapple (forthcoming) observes that even palliative care can, at times, be end-oriented, dominated by the clock time of the hospital, and hurried.

There are, however, cases in which definitions of cure are more nuanced in contemporary biomedicine. An example of this can be seen in the treatment of cancer. Knowing that complete eradication is hard to determine, success in cancer treatment is measured in five year survival rates. Also, in advanced cases of cancer, doctors try to weigh the benefits of abrasive therapies against the patient's "quality of life," the degree of mental and psychological suffering he/she is undergoing.[4] More pertinent to this study, schizophrenia is often considered to be a chronic problem "characterized by remissions and relapses," and a variety of outcomes, such as "occupational functioning and social competence," are considered.[5] In addition, some people undergo psychotherapy as an ongoing process of self exploration and development rather than simply to cure or overcome a problem. Still, some researchers in biomedicine have recently questioned the emphasis on curing and would like to see palliative care extended to a wider variety of problems, not only illnesses that are deemed incurable. They critique an emphasis on cure that obscures other goals of treatment and consideration of how painful it is to undergo a course of therapy.[6]

Medical historians Jecker and Self (1991) suggest that in the past greater attention was paid to care and palliation which changed with biomedicine's attempts to gain prestige and develop as a profession. A division between care and cure resulted in part from competition with homeopathic healers and lay people, often relatives, who nursed–that is, took care of—the ill, which was considered women's work and devalued. Jecker and Self conclude:

> The early history of American medicine suggests a possible explanation for the association of medicine with cure, rather than care. The presence of fierce competition and marginal status during its early years forged a mission for medicine that focused on achieving cultural authority and an elite status for its practitioners. Efforts to gain authority and status required physicians to stand apart from laypersons and develop exclusive modes of language, technique and theory. This put physicians at odds with activities, such as patient empathy and care, that call upon abilities of engagement and identification with others (293).

I would add that the issues Jecker and Self discuss are more acute when the dis-ease involves a psychological and emotional pathology. While people are normally willing to endure unpleasant and curatively-oriented procedures for problems that are more acute and more firmly rooted in the body—and this includes people in India (Van Hollen 2003)—treatment that involves aesthetic discomfort and pain is more problematic when the mind, emotion or self are afflicted.

Reactions to Ayurveda and Allopathy

In Chapter 1, Ajit, the young man who was undergoing therapy with an ayurvedic psychiatrist and had formerly been treated by allopathic psychiatrists, introduced us to some of the differences, as he saw them, between allopathic and ayurvedic psychiatric treatments:

> I came to [name of allopathic hospital], took "injection"s and was given a new medicine. Later I was forced to stop it. The reason was that I had started

shivering. [. . .] In the case of allopathic doctors, after asking two or three questions, they will know which medicine to prescribe. But ayurvedic doctors, they want to take the patient to another level. At that level, things are very different. Right now I am taking treatment for mental illness. For this illness, there is a painful method. It is giving electric "shock"s. After going there [allopathy] and coming here [ayurveda], I feel this is better.

One sees in this excerpt frequently-heard complaints about uncomfortable effects of medications and electroconvulsive therapy in allopathic psychiatry. Ajit says injections of medications caused him to start shivering, and he describes "electric shocks" as a "painful method" of treatment. This passage also contains an enthusiastic evaluation of ayurvedic care. Some patients undergoing treatment that involved what I call a pleasant process also enthusiastically described their treatment not only as a way of getting rid of a problem but also as a means of transformation—or, as Ajit put it, bringing one to "another level." This is not to imply that patients did not see benefits to allopathic care. Allopathy has its own virtues—such as obtaining fast results as we shall see later—but these did not include pleasant or "cooling" experiences or the possibility of achieving "another level" of health.

Reactions to Electroconvulsive Therapy and Talapodichil

Working just South of Kerala in Sri Lanka, Nichter and Nordstrom (1989) observed that people perceive allopathy as a powerful and "heating" medicine that can give quick relief but can also cause serious side effects:

Allopathic medicines are spoken of as "shocking" the body and causing side effects which may prove as troublesome as those symptoms originally prompting one to seek treatment (Nichter and Nordstrom 1989: 374).

The illustrations that follow reveal a situation where shocking the body is more than a metaphor for allopathic treatment. A comparison of patient reactions to the allopathic inpatient psychiatric procedure electroconvulsive therapy and the ayurvedic inpatient psychiatric procedure known as *talapodichil* reveals how a powerful and "shocking" therapy feels and demonstrates the importance of a pleasant process of treatment for people undergoing therapy.

Electroconvulsive therapy (or ECT—also known as "shock therapy" or "electroshock therapy") involves sending an electrical current through a patient's body at a level high enough to cause a seizure. This procedure is used in inpatient allopathic psychiatric treatment in Kerala for acutely suicidal patients, severely depressed patients and psychotic patients who do not respond to medications. These are generally the same conditions under which ECT is used in the U.S., although issues discussed in this section may be more acute in India where, some evidence suggests, ECT is administered more frequently.[7] For several informants I spoke with in Kerala, aversion to ECT was a significant factor in deciding to discontinue allopathic psychiatric care and pursue another form of therapy.

I felt it was too intrusive to directly observe ECT sessions in India. In fact, the awkwardness of doing so and the ease of observing the ayurvedic treatment sessions—ECT occurring behind closed doors and the ayurvedic therapies being administered in open view of other patients and visitors—reinforces the distinctions highlighted in this comparison of treatment procedures. My information on ECT comes from patient accounts and my glimpses of preparations for ECT and its aftermath. Patients who are awaiting treatment at the Trivandrum Medical College hospital sit on a bench in the hospital out-patient area (OP). The only aesthetic or visceral experience patients engage with before ECT perhaps comes from the institutional facility of the psychiatric OP itself. As suggested earlier, the effort to avoid aesthetic engagement and create a sterile environment has the unintended consequence of creating the feel and smell of a hospital which is not necessarily unpleasant but does not actively engage patients with a positive aesthetic experience. The rooms of the psychiatric OP are stark, and, if decorated, apparently haphazardly so, with usually nothing more than an official government calendar on the wall. There is nothing to actively engage the senses other than watching the comings and goings of other patients. After the administration of the electric currents and undergoing seizures, which are meant to be therapeutic, patients have completed ECT and are wheeled out on a gurney looking catatonic or unconscious, attached to an intravenous catheter, while family members who were waiting for the patient appeared sober and concerned. This contrasted with the demeanor of patients following *talapodichil*.

Kuttappan is a 64 year-old Hindu man who was undergoing the 45-day *panchakarma* treatment at the Government Ayurveda Mental Hospital (GAMH) having previously tried allopathy for problems that included crying and talking too much, showing too much anger and talking nonsensically. These problems started three or four years earlier after a horrible tragedy where Kuttappan's daughter-in-law killed her son and then herself. He was originally treated at an allopathic hospital, and his condition improved. Recently, however, his illness returned, and Kuttappan's wife, who was taking care of him at the GAMH, explained that they decided not to return to an allopathic hospital because of fear of the effect of ECT on her somewhat elderly husband:

> They told us we should take him to [name of allopathic hospital]. He is old now. If we take him there, they'll give him a shock or something. He is 64 years old. Here they give only native medicine and will get change [*māttam*]. They [some relatives] told us there was improvement [*bhēdam*] with this medicine for their son so we took him here. He has a cough and asthma now, but he will get over it. This treatment can do all this.

On a previous visit to an allopathic hospital, Kuttappan ran away from the hospital claiming the staff was doing black magic on him. I do not know if this was a reaction to ECT or other aspects of treatment or if he was given ECT during his first stay at the allopathic hospital. I did not specifically enquire about this because I was not specifically looking for reactions to ECT when we met Kuttappan.

In addition to her worries about allopathic treatment, Kuttappan's wife's statement reveals a degree of enthusiasm in describing their expectations and experience in ayurvedic care. I heard several enthusiastic descriptions among other ayurvedic patients and persons using religious therapies, but such descriptions were rare among patients we interviewed who were using allopathic medicine. Some patients say they were helped by allopathy, some say they appreciated the quick effects of allopathic treatment, but interviewees did not offer nostalgic or enthusiastic descriptions of allopathic care. Also, Kuttappan's wife uses the term *māttam*, which best translates as "change," and *bhēdam* which means "improvement," to describe what they hope to accomplish in seeking therapy. Neither of these terms, nor indeed any term in Malayalam used for the dispensation of an illness has the remedial, return-to-normalcy implications inherent in the concept of "cure."[8] They leave open the possibility of more modest or more exalted forms of "change" than what is implied by "curing" or "healing."

In discussing the outcome of an earlier stay at an allopathic hospital with my assistant Benny, Kuttappan's wife recalled:

> Kuttappan's Wife: After staying there, the problem was gone [literally, "there was nothing" *onnum undāyilla*].

> Benny: After taking treatment from there he was completely okay [*pournamāyi sariyāyi*].

> Kuttappan's Wife: After 22 days, all of his illnesses had changed/were gone [*ellā asukhavum māri*].

It is possible to interpret these three ways of talking about the outcome of Kuttappan's treatment as approximations of the concept of "cure" as complete eradication of a problem—although it is difficult to say whether a return to normalcy is implied. It is probably significant that these efforts to speak of something like complete change or complete absence occur in the context of discussing allopathic care. Unfortunately, Kuttappan's problems did return after "all of his illnesses had changed" following allopathic therapy. Kuttappan's wife's expectations about ayurvedic therapy probably also remained unfulfilled since we learned from reviewing medical records on a follow-up visit to the GAMH that Kuttappan had been released before completing therapy. We never learned exactly why he was released early. He may have reacted in a paranoid manner to the staff, as he did in allopathic treatment, and left voluntarily. Or he may have been released because of violent outbursts that occurred while he was staying at the GAMH.

Mathew John, a 35-year-old Christian man, was being treated at the GAMH accompanied by his father. Benny and I interviewed Mathew John and his father later in the course of field research after I had begun to notice complaints about unpleasant treatments and became interested in reactions to allopathic therapy. Mathew John's comments should be viewed in the context that Benny and I were explicitly asking Mathew John to evaluate his allopathic treatment. After hearing general, unspecified complaints about allopathic therapy from several patients, we felt it would be appropriate to ask Mathew John specifically what he did not like about allopathic treatment:

Benny: What kind of treatment did you receive in allopathy?

Mathew John and Father (together): They gave ECT five times plus tablets and injections.

Benny: Did you like allopathy?

Mathew John: I didn't like it.

Benny: What specifically didn't you like?

Mathew John: I didn't like ECT.

Mathew John had been hearing sounds, and he was afraid he was being pursued by evil spirits and people who were trying to hurt him. He had a good income as a clerk in a public school, but his pathologies undermined his ability to work. His family sought treatment at an allopathic hospital when his problem first emerged in 1989, and he was hospitalized in allopathic institutions four times before coming to the GAMH.

Abdul Aziz is a 27 year-old man who was receiving treatment at the GAMH. He was accompanied by his father who told us that he had been talking incoherently and had been violent. Abdul Aziz also had itching and pain in his body which he said were caused by a spirit. During three years of allopathic psychiatric treatment, he received ECT nine times and took as many as 16 pills a day. Abdul Aziz' father also explained that the "head treatment" at the GAMH made Abdul Aziz feel "cool and calm." In my meetings with him, Abdul Aziz was pleasant, upbeat and eccentric, and he was often wearing the mudpack and banana leaf of *talapodichil* treatment.

Whereas no patients said they enjoyed the effects of ECT and some recalled this as an uncomfortable or painful procedure, several patients described positive aesthetic reactions to *talapodichil* and other ayurvedic treatments. A number of inpatient ayurvedic procedures could be compared to ECT. *Talapodichil* is the most well-known and high profile inpatient psychiatric procedure in ayurveda much like ECT's standing within allopathic treatment, and in this sense it is an appropriate procedure for comparison. Also, what will be said below about *talapodichil* is generally true of the other ayurvedic inpatient psychiatric treatments I investigated at GAMH in the sense that informants report they cause little discomfort or are aesthetically pleasing. What Abdul Aziz' father refers to as "head treatment" is most likely *talapodichil* although he could be referring to *pichu*, which involves applying medicated oil to the head (described in Chapter 2) and, according to patients, is an equally "cooling" therapy. "Cooling" describes a physiologically or aesthetically pleasant effect based on lay South Asian views of health and aesthetics.

I will always associate Abdul Aziz with *talapodichil*. On one of my first visits to the GAMH, as I walked up the steps to the verandah of the traditional Malabar mansion that had been converted into the ayurvedic mental hospital, Abdul Aziz approached me, the top of his head wrapped with a banana leaf concealing the *talapodichil* mudpack he was wearing. He smiled, pumped my hand enthusiastically and welcomed me to the hospital. In subsequent visits, Abdul Aziz continued to enthusiastically welcome me, and I was charmed by this tall, comical figure who on more than one occasion I saw marching around the hospital with the banana leaf on his head singing "la illaha il allah" (an Arabic phrase meaning "there is no god but Allah"). Although not every patient was as outgoing as Abdul Aziz, whether it was due to the "cooling" effect of the therapy or the comical look of the banana leaf "hat," people who were undergoing *talapodichil* were usually in a good humor, and their demeanor contrasted sharply with that of patients who were preparing for or had recently undergone a round of ECT.

After completing four weeks of *panchakarma* treatment, which includes taking purgatives, enemas and nasally-administered medicines while on a special vegetarian diet (described in more detail in Chapter 2), the patient at the GAMH receives *talapodichil*.[9]

Talapodichil is performed, along with other ayurvedic procedures, in the late afternoon on the outdoor verandah of the GAMH.[10] The patient who is to receive *talapodichil* sits on the short wall of the verandah. A nurse unwraps what I have been calling a "mudpack," a ball of ayurvedic *materia medica* including *nellikka* (gooseberry) and yogurt curd, which resembles wet earth or clay. The nurse removes and puts aside a small portion of the "mud," then rubs oil on the patient's head (which, if the patient is male, has been shaved), and molds the large portion of the mud onto the patient's head from the top of the skull down to the top of the forehead and about as far down on the back and sides. A banana leaf is then tied over the mudpack to keep it in place, and the patient is allowed to walk around the hospital compound or relax, as he or she wishes. (See Figures 4 and 5 which show nurses administering *talapodichil* to a patient at the GAMH.) After 45 minutes, the patient returns to the treatment area, and a portion of mud is removed from an area between the forehead and the top of the skull that is considered an important center of mental activity. The mud removed from this area, which physicians at the hospital say will have warmed to a temperature around 40° Celsius, is replaced with the small portion of mud that was set aside at the beginning of the procedure. After another 45 minutes, the mudpack and banana leaf are completely removed and the patient wanders off to socialize or relax.

People I spoke with who were undergoing *talapodichil* said it had a cooling effect on their head and body. One patient joked that it was like having an "AC" (i.e., Air-Conditioned) hat. Ajit, the former patient of the GAMH who was introduced earlier, reflecting on his treatment there recalled: "I got some more energy, especially a little improvement in 'memory.' My head got cooled." "Cooling" (*tanuppa, kulirmma* and other terms) is a cultural idiom for a pleasant physical, visceral state or effect. In many parts of South Asia, there is a lay (non-specialist, though loosely related to ayurveda) system of classification of foods, weather, times of day, emotions and many other things as heating or cooling. Mental imbalance is often, though not always, considered to be due to excess heat that affects the head and can be countered by substances and circumstances that create cooling effects.[11] However, cooling has many meanings beyond the realm of mental disorder. It can refer to a pleasant aesthetic effect in many contexts. People in Kerala—friends, research assistants and others—were often telling me what would give one a cooling effect: from drinking salt with your lime juice, to building your home a certain way, to visiting certain parts of a

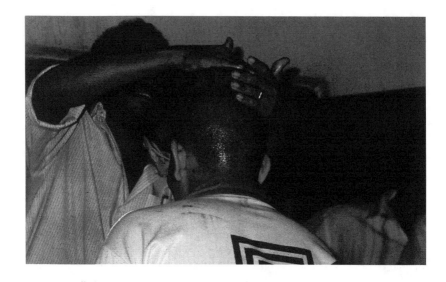

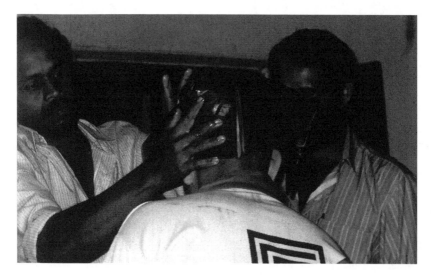

Figures 4 and 5. Nurses administering *talapodichil* to a patient at the Government Ayurveda Mental Hospital.

temple. Ajit also used the word *kulirmma* to describe what one can attain from ayurveda. *Kulirmma* can be translated as "coolness," "freshness," "satisfaction" or "delight," indicating, in line with Kerala's phenomenological orientation, a broader meaning than just physical pleasure or comfort.

Reactions to Medications

Another, more frequently heard set of complaints several ayurvedic patients brought up regarding their previous allopathic treatment concerned the effects of allopathic medications.

A 30-year-old Hindu man, Raju, had been having problems ever since he returned during the 1991 Gulf War from Kuwait where he had been working as a mechanic. He had had violent outbursts, he would laugh without reason, and he threatened to destroy his family's property. Raju's mother, who accompanied him while he was being treated at the GAMH, explained that allopathic medicines were unpleasant and made him tired which led Raju and his family to change therapies:

> We changed from allopathy to ayurveda because he felt tired from allopathic treatment. He didn't like the effects of allopathic medicines. They made him feel tired. He felt allopathic treatment caused memory loss.

Bindu, a 36-year-old Hindu woman who was receiving treatment at the GAMH had a similar reaction to allopathic (which she calls "English") medications. Bindu had been depressed and "lost mental control" when she attacked her brother's wife and his son. She was sent to an allopathic psychiatrist, but she changed to ayurvedic therapy because allopathic medications made her feel sluggish and tired:

> English medicines made me too tired. I couldn't even respond when spoken to. I felt less tired with ayurvedic medicine. I felt weight in my head during English medicine which is now gone.

We interviewed 26-year-old Mohammed Koya and several of his relatives after they consulted with an ayurvedic psychiatrist about admitting Mohammed to the GAMH. Mohammed had returned from working as a waiter in the Persian Gulf because of his illness which has a variety of manifestations including laughing for no reason, anger toward his family and refusing to leave home to go to work. Mohammed's relatives told us that he had been to an allopathic hospital and was taking allopathic medications. He could function on these medications, but they made him tired and he did not want to have to take pills all his life, which an allopathic psychiatrist said would be necessary. The family decided to pursue ayurvedic treatment because they had heard that through ayurveda one could get off pills. This perception does reflect the practices at the GAMH. Patients who are already taking allopathic medicines when admitted are slowly weaned off these medications over the initial period of treatment.

I used the same interview questions and format with allopathic patients, but, even if they had positive reactions about other aspects of allopathic therapy, they did not offer any positive evaluations of the aesthetic experience of undergoing allopathic treatment. For example, no allopathic treatment was described as "cooling." When patients said something good about allopathy it was usually that they experienced improvement in their condition. This is not to say that more patients experienced improvement with allopathy. An evaluation of short term (six to nine month) outcomes among patients of allopathy, ayurveda and religious therapies showed no significant difference between these three therapies in terms of effectiveness at improving patients' conditions although certain therapies appeared more appropriate for certain patients.[12] For example, an engineering student we interviewed at an allopathic hospital was the most fervent supporter of allopathy which he praised for being "more logical, more methodical." Also, while several Muslim patients say they benefited from healing at Beemapalli mosque, a Muslim woman whose husband is an army nurse, and who said she did not believe in religious healing, felt she experienced no improvement from visiting Beemapalli but got relief through allopathic care.

Regarding the aesthetic process of healing, a few allopathic patients also offered complaints about unpleasant effects of allopathic therapies that resembled those reported by ayurvedic patients reflecting on allopathic treatment. A young man, Varghese, who was seeking treatment at an allopathic facility when we spoke to him recalled the treatment he received earlier at another allopathic facility:

> I was taken to [name of hospital]. There I was given three shocks. I felt numbness in my head when I got the first shock. [. . .] There I completed six months of treatment, I broke my lips [he later explained that this was due to ECT], was totally tired mentally, and came home. I could not write my examination in maths. [. . .] I was given an injection. Terrible pain. When I requested to do counseling, I was called in and examined for swelling.

Varghese's way of avoiding these uncomfortable effects of therapy was to seek treatment at the allopathic facility he was currently utilizing but from a clinical psychologist who relied on fewer medications.

Some people who were using religious therapies had similar evaluations of the aesthetics of allopathic therapy. The wife of Hanifa the former Gulf migrant introduced in Chapter 3, who was seeking relief for his "tension" and sleeplessness at Beemapalli mosque, was concerned about memory problems her husband experienced from taking allopathic psychiatric medications:

Kavitha: Are you taking "allopathy" medicine now?

Wife: No, no.

Kavitha: Now he is not taking any medicine.

Murphy: Now it is finished.

Wife: Now that he is not taking medicine, there is a lot of improvement. When he was taking medicine, he had memory problems [literally, reduction—*kuravu*].

[...]

Kavitha: Was it because of memory problems that you stopped, or ...?

Wife: Yeah, because of memory problems and a lot of "tension," thinking, and he was like this. So we changed. Now there is relief after coming here. After he came here, he sleeps without taking medicine.

A quantitative analysis of the aesthetic evaluations of treatment in allopathy and ayurveda among all informants yielded the following overview:

- 95 of the patients my assistants and I interviewed were currently using or had previously tried allopathy. A total of 14 of these informants offered, without our asking, some complaint about the effect of psychiatric medications or ECT during their allopathic treatment.
- 42 patients interviewed were currently using or had previously tried ayurveda. None complained of abrasive effects of ayurvedic therapy though some said ayurvedic treatment could be "difficult" to undergo.

Another way to interpret patients' visceral reactions to treatment is to compare the aesthetics of adversity in ayurveda and allopathy. As mentioned earlier, not all ayurvedic treatments are "pleasant." There is the discomfort of drinking *snehapana* (ghee for oleation of the body) and undergoing *vamana* (drinking a purgative to remove impurities from the body through emesis). One ayurvedic patient said ayurveda was more difficult to undergo than allopathy, and he explained this "difficulty" in terms of the lengthiness of treatments one had to endure in ayurvedic therapy which he contrasted to the quick and simple administrations of allopathic injections. Another similarly contrasted the discipline and regimen of ayurvedic therapy (which at the GAMH, where he was being treated, requires 45 days of inpatient treatment and dietary restrictions) with the quick treatment of allopathy. Yet another patient explained that ayurvedic therapy was difficult because it was hard to drink ghee (referring to the *snehapana* treatment which was described as akin to the discomfort of eating too much heavy food) and he did not like having to give up smoking and eating meat while in treatment. However, he added that after a while he began to feel good on this more austere, vegetarian regimen. Allopathy, by contrast, may be seen as creating at times sharp, heating unpleasant effects, a different kind of abrasiveness. Perhaps the difference is that allopathy's effects are unintended, "side effects" as many in Kerala point out, and it may be that the sense of inappropriate or unexpected effects—as opposed to the expectation of discomfort and inconvenience in some ayurvedic panchakarma procedures— causes a more adverse reaction, exacerbating the somatic-aesthetic experience in allopathic treatment.

The most significant difference, however, is that while both allopathic and ayurvedic procedures feature unpleasant or challenging effects, only ayurvedic treatment included therapies that were reported as actually pleasant or "cooling" to undergo. No allopathic therapy inspired positive aesthetic appraisals. No patient explained that they enjoyed undergoing injections or ECT, even though some said they benefited from these therapies.

There are certainly contexts in India and other parts of the world where there is a sense of "pleasure" in pain or redemptive effects of suffering, but there was little indication of such an orientation among people suffering psychopathology in Kerala. The "difficulty" in undergoing the lengthy and— especially for those who normally smoke, drink alcohol or eat meat—austere regimen was recounted with a sense of bravado, a certain sense of pleasure or pride in overcoming a challenge, but there was no articulation among patients of a sense that pain or discomfort was necessary for healing, or at least for healing problems of *manas* and *bōdham*.

Displeasure or pain is an important part of the process in other contexts in South India, for example, in particular rituals and pilgrimages. On a road near the Medical College campus in Trivandrum as I was on my way to meet an allopathic psychiatrist, I observed a *taipooja* ritual wherein devotees pierce their lower lips with long skewers and parade down the street in a demonstration of devotion to the divine marked, in part, by overcoming or enduring the discomfort of the piercing. Daniel (1984) famously depicted his own experience among Tamil pilgrims who were undertaking a 40 kilometer trek to the Sabarimala shrine in the mountains of Kerala. Walking barefoot on rocky, blazing hot trails, Daniel describes the experience of increasing pain which devotees struggle to defy in order to enhance their devotion to the deity Aiyappan. Daniel recalls being able to distinguish between the pain in different parts of his feet and the pain in his shoulders and head, distinctions which are eventually replaced by a generalized feeling of pain. Finally, through this experience the ego is obscured and replaced by what Daniel explains as an experience of Peircean Firstness and the devotees claim is an immediate realization of love for the deity (266–270). Such painful trials were not expected or undertaken by people I spoke with who underwent religious therapies at Chottanikkara, Beemapalli or Vettucaud. Perhaps this is because they were already suffering. Their primary sensory engagements came through singing devotional songs, smelling incense, engaging visually with a dramatic outdoor setting (recall the location of Vettucaud church on the beach and the evocative architecture of the religious settings), praying as the sun rises and feeling the cool stone of the temple walkways under their bare feet. As a counterpart to Daniel's own pain, and reward, of participating in the Sabarimala pilgrimage, I enjoyed the aesthetic engagements I experienced in visiting religious healing sites and following the mentally afflicted through their routines.[13] Indeed, my assistants and I most preferred visiting religious centers when we set out to conduct interviews and observations. The spacious grounds and ornamental architecture of these settings provided a visceral sense of relief from the crowded busy spaces of the Indian city that we usually inhabited.

In a different medical context in nearby Tamil Nadu, Van Hollen (2003) shows how women in childbirth demand oxytocin drugs, which speed the labor process but cause more painful contractions. However, these women do not take anesthetics since they feel the pain they experience is necessary for the proper delivery of their child. Furthermore, Tamil women derive their *sakti*, a sense of power that is associated with femaleness, in part from their "ability to suffer nobly the pain of birth" (58). The administration of pain-relieving drugs would thus rob them of their sakti, and Van Hollen adds that "some women went so far as to say that the oxytocin-induced pain *increased* their sakti" (58). Thus, in the case of treatments for psychopathology in Kerala and the medical management of childbirth in Tamil Nadu, allopathic treatments are experienced as abrasive or painful. But while this experience leads some mentally afflicted patients in Kerala to pursue other, gentler treatment options, the experience of pain leads Tamil women to refuse (or in some cases make a virtue of the scarcity of) pain reducing drugs. It may be that in the medical context, for conditions that are more fully of the body, discomfort is more acceptable while for problems that affect more intangible parts of the person, such as *manas* and *bōdham*, abrasive aesthetic experiences are less acceptable.[14]

This comparison between allopathic and ayurvedic treatments should be qualified with the observation that the distinction between more abrasive therapies in allopathy and gentler therapies in ayurveda was not always clear. In the past, treatments were used in ayurveda that were more analogous to ECT. Dr. Rajendra Varma of the Vaidyarathnam Oushadhasala ayurvedic clinic explained that "in the olden days," "instead of this psychiatric treatment—shock treatment—we used to take the patient to the execution room and we would bring in an elephant and ask the elephant just to show its leg as if to squeeze the head, to press the head of the patient." The elephant would raise its leg over the patient's head as if to crush it. The patient would become frightened, and then the elephant's leg would be removed. Alternately, Dr. Varma said uniformed men would drag the patient before the king who would accuse the patient of a crime and demand that he be executed. The trial would then be revealed as a hoax. These procedures are also described, along with suggestions to beat patients with certain kinds of mental illnesses, in the classical ayurvedic medical text *Caraka Samhita* (1998: 436–437 [Cikitsāsthānam, Ch. IX, Verses 79–84]).

Francis Zimmermann's (1992) analysis of what he refers to as the contemporary "flower power of ayurveda" claims that abrasive therapies have been discontinued in modern ayurvedic practice as ayurveda redefines an identity for itself in relation to allopathic medicine. Classical ayurveda, Zimmermann explains, featured some violent and cathartic procedures, but in the context of competition with allopathy—recognizing that allopathy has essentially cornered the market on invasive procedures such as surgery—ayurveda emphasizes the balanced, gentle and nonviolent aspects of its practice.

Addressing the government of Travancore (the colonial princely state that later formed the southern portion of Kerala) in 1926 to contest the fact that the state's Ayurveda Department was receiving much less funding than the Allopathy Department, T. K. Velupillai argued that: "Although, Allopathic medicines are powerful and useful, Ayurvedic medicines are found to be keeping with our mode of life (sic)." The meaning of this is a little cryptic, but later he added "Europeans live on beef, ham, apricots and champagne. They have the habit of smoking cigarette. But we live on rice, tapioca [a starchy root vegetable], pickles and perhaps a little milk or buttermilk. We have the habit of taking oil bath (sic)" (quoted in Nair 2001: 228). This may have been part of an effort to highlight the "gentle" nature of ayurveda in the face of the growing influence of allopathy, which at the time had strong support from the colonial and princely governments, Christian missionaries and the Rockefeller Foundation. In his association between allopathic medicine and European culinary habits Velupillai mentions beef and alcohol which, like allopathic medicines, are seen as "heating," a quality which can be dangerous, destabilizing and adverse to mental health. Velupillai emphasizes the vegetarian nature of the local diet (referring even guiltily to taking "perhaps a little" milk and buttermilk which are considered only marginally vegetarian) and refers to taking oil baths, which are akin to the *picchu* treatment patients at the GAMH found aesthetically agreeable. Many people in Kerala today do eat meat and fish and also smoke and drink, but recall that patients at the GAMH were required to give up these indulgences while undergoing treatment.

Regardless of whether the emphasis on gentleness is a modern or (post) colonial innovation, it is something that clients of ayurveda appreciate. This is perhaps a case of effective maneuvering around the hegemony, in terms of funding and government support, of allopathic medicine. Ayurveda emphasized nonviolent approaches to health and illness and attracted some patients away from allopathy. Or it may have been the case that ayurvedic practitioners realized that in relation to allopathy they need to emphasize what they do best, to promote practices that they felt were more unique to ayurveda. It is possible that ayurveda never developed or emphasized invasive interventions for acute problems in the way that allopathy did. Several healers and non-medical specialists in Kerala depicted allopathic medicine as more appropriate for acute and traumatic illness and injury while claiming that ayurveda excels at treating chronic problems that take time to develop and to treat. Indeed, as we will see later, the speed of onset of a problem and the speed of the process of therapy are reshaping some people's relations to these two medical practices.

Thus healing systems continually realign in relation to one another, which is not to say that they are merely constructed or lacking in unique features of knowledge and practice. And this type of readjustment in this medically plural environment is not new. While in the colonial and postcolonial period, ayurveda and allopathy, and their promoters, react to each other, in an earlier period, ayurvedic practitioners adapted methods from the Islamically-associated unani medicine in north India (Leslie 1976). While healers are influenced by, or resist, other medical practices, people with illnesses who navigate these systems respond to and call for realignments, as we saw in the case of patients who discontinued allopathic psychiatric care because of concerns about unpleasant or dangerous effects of treatment. These patients basically vote with their feet, which is something that occurs more often in a medically plural society, and can have an impact on the nature of medical practice.[15] Allopathic practitioners might be tempted to reinvent their practice to emphasize more gentle treatments, but they may be concerned that allopathy might lose its distinction as a fast, invasive, and, at times, heroic medicine, especially for acute and infectious cases.

A Pleasant Process as Resolution and
Enhanced States of "Health"

The significance of the pleasantness of the treatment process extends beyond the issue of the relative pleasantness or abrasiveness of undergoing treatment. Some patients remained in a pleasant, aesthetically-engaging healing process as a "solution" to an intractable problem while others recalled their process of healing with enthusiasm and described a movement to a state that was more auspicious, somehow more enhanced or more vibrant than the state of health that existed before their illness.

How does one continue with a mental affliction if one has been pursuing treatment for this problem for years, going in and out of allopathic and ayurvedic psychiatric hospitals, having tried homeopathic medicine, *mantravādam* (magic), and other measures? At what point does constant "treatment" become a burden? Some mentally afflicted people my research assistants and I spoke to had been living at a temple, mosque or church for years, having previously tried more medically-oriented treatments for several years. These individuals had reached a point where engaging in a pleasant process, living in the pleasant, aesthetically- and spiritually-engaging environment of a temple, mosque or church, itself became a way of managing their problems.

Sasi is a Hindu man in his late twenties who is possessed and has been living at Beemapalli mosque with his mother for years after spending a good portion of his life trying other treatments. Sasi has exhibited a variety of problematic behaviors related to his possession by several spirits including attacking family members, running away from home, and refusing to speak for days at a time. Eight and a half years before our interview, when his problems started, Sasi's family went to see a *mantravādan*, a specialist in magic, to counter sorcery which Sasi's mother said was likely the cause of his affliction. Sasi then spent a year in inpatient and outpatient treatment at a private allopathic psychiatric hospital and two years in a state allopathic psychiatric hospital. For the last five years, he has been at Beemapalli mosque, and his mother says that it is only at Beemapalli that there is "change" in his illness. During a follow-up interview seven months after our original interview, Sasi and his mother were still at Beemapalli and Sasi's mother told us that Sasi's condition has been "up and down." She said she believes one gets relief by going through ups and downs, and affirmed that she and her son "have complete faith in Beemapalli."

Kavitha and I spoke with Mustapha, a Muslim fisherman in his mid-forties, and his younger brother who was staying with him while he sought relief for his problems at Beemapalli mosque. Recalling a long and seemingly fruitless course of therapy-seeking, Mustapha's brother explained:

> This is the fifth time it has come. The problem has been coming and going for the past eight to ten years. We don't go anywhere else now. We took him everywhere and lost a lot of money and he didn't get better [lit. "didn't become healthy"— *sukhamāvilla*]. When we take him here, he becomes healthy [*sukhamāvunnuntu*]. This time we came here three months ago.

[...]

> We are giving him no medicine other than that. Now there is some relief [lit. "lessening/reduction"—*kuravu*]. He will get some relief during these months. We are sure about it.

Kavitha: When he is sick, how long do you have to stay here?

Brother: Until he gets relief. Now it won't take more than two months.

Mustapha had been hitting and swearing at anyone who came near him while also talking strangely and exhibiting other symptoms of disturbance. Since his problems first emerged 23 years ago after failing his Secondary School Leaving Exam, he was treated at a state-run allopathic psychiatric hospital where he received ECT. His family also tried *mantravādam* (magic, to counter sorcery), but the only place where he got relief was at Beemapalli:

> Now when we take him to this mosque, he will get relief. Like that, nine years ago we took him straight here. We did not try any other place at that time. Wherever else we have gone there is no improvement. We will spend money but whatever hospital we go to, whatever *mantravādan* we see, he won't get relief. At last, after having spent all our money on his treatment, we will take him here and here he will get relief.

Mustapha's problems have, of course, resurfaced, and he has spent the last six weeks at Beemapalli. Our conversation with his brother shows that his family has resolved to live with this recurring problem and occasionally seek "some relief" and "reduction" through visits to the mosque.

Mariyamma is an elderly Christian woman who lives at Vettucaud church, the beachfront Catholic church and healing center in Trivandrum. Mariyamma has been taking allopathic medicines for the last six years for sleeping and breathing problems related to family tensions. She also prays at Vettucaud church to find relief from her affliction. This should not be taken to mean that Mariyamma is praying to find some future relief for her problems, though that may happen. Her prayers, at this spiritually auspicious and aesthetically engaging setting on the Arabian Sea, *are* her relief at present. When asked what future plans she has to cope with her problems, Mariyamma explained, "I want to remain here until the end of my life."

Mariyamma, Mustapha, Sasi and others like them are managing their problems and pursuing the modest goals of relief, reduction or change through living periodically, or on a continuing basis, in the aesthetically and spiritually engaging environments of religious healing centers. No interviewees developed such place relations to other healing centers. No one chose to live on the campus of the allopathic Medical College Hospital or the Government Ayurveda Mental Hospital periodically as a way of coping with recurring problems. Indeed, it is not possible to do so at these settings although patients may have visited healing centers such as these on repeated occasions in undergoing multiple courses of treatment. This analysis is not meant to imply that people who have resigned to live with an intractable problem would not later be open to the possibility of radical changes, complete cures or transformative improvements in their lives and problems, but it appears that after years of actively pursuing treatments for their problems, some individuals have de-emphasized the contingency of time in relating to their illness and resolved to seek occasional relief for a recurring problem at a religious center.

Such dispositions are not unknown in allopathic psychiatry. Despite efforts to work toward the ideal of achieving a cure, some problems are considered essentially incurable or chronic. Those diagnosed as schizophrenic, for example, are often seen as requiring long term, even life-long, pharmaceutical management and move in an out of psychiatric institutions over the course of many years (Estroff 1981)—and it would not be hard to imagine that Sasi and Mustapha might have received such diagnoses during their allopathic treatment. It appears that Sasi, Mustapha and Mariyamma have found a more "pleasant" alternative to a life of institutional management or repeated, unpleasant attempts at achieving a cure. They and their family caretakers speak of modest and incremental moments of relief, change and reduction which they accomplish by essentially living in a pleasant process of therapy in the spiritually and aesthetically engaging environment of a mosque, temple or church. While these idioms of incremental relief stop short of the English language/allopathic ideal of "curing," other idioms speak of experiences that transcend the restorative, return to pre-illness state goals of allopathic care.

Rajan was the young man introduced in Chapter 2 who was formerly possessed at Chottanikkara temple and was so affected by his "healing" experience that he decided to live at the temple and work at the temple lodge. His description of his possession-healing experience was spirited, nostalgic, and recounted with a you-have-to-try-it-for-yourself tone. Rajan's depiction of the daily routine of afflicted devotees provides a sense of the color, variety, and opportunities for sensory engagement as well as his own enthusiasm toward devotional healing practices at Chottanikkara (although his excited description in Malayalam, laced with English terms and Sanskritic Hindu religious terminology, does not translate smoothly):

> The "first" *bhajan* [devotional singing] starts at 3:30 am. Then the "temple" will be open at 4. Then there are the remaining demi-gods: Ayappan, Sivan, Murugan, Ganapathy, Sarppan. It will open "completely", then we will walk around the temple. Then there are *pūjas* [worships/offerings/encounters] and consecrations. There will be *dhāra* [a sprinkling of water ritual] at the Siva shrine. Then almost at the same time, it will start. We will start shaking like this [the possessing spirit will become active]. It will start at five o'clock in the morning. Then at eight we have ghee. After that, we will have fruit or something. We are not allowed to eat any food prepared outside. *Naivēdyam* [an offering of food to the deities before being eaten by worshippers] will be done at noon. That food will be the meal we eat in the afternoon. Have you seen *kuruti* [a worship invoking the goddess Kali]? You will see *kuruti pūja* tonight.

The devotional routine for those suffering affliction thus engages the sense— aural, kinaesthetic and gustatory in this case. They start the day with singing followed by pre-dawn rituals at the temple and sharing of food with the deities. At the end of the excerpt, Rajan is excited that my assistant Biju and I should see what is essentially part of the healing process, the *kuruti* ceremony. After mentioning *kuruti*, Rajan's description moves to the beginning of the next day:

> Then we are ready to go again at 4 am. We will bathe again, become "fresh" and will go to the temple. After bathing, we will walk around the temple. There are four *pūjas*. At 6 o'clock is *dīparādhana* [waving lamps in front of an idol], *śīveli* is at 7 o'clock. At 8:30 at night, *kuruti* begins again. It will be over at 9:30. Thus "full time" we are in this temple or under its "treatment." We will not know anything about what is going on outside. "Full concentration, full prayer." We will be "fully" praying. [. . .] we chant the *Saraswatham* [for the goddess Saraswati] and *Garudarudam* [for Vishnu] mantras and the Garuda *panchakāra* [a hymn]. We enter while chanting these mantras. These mantras have a good relationship with nature. They will make us "pure automatically."

In addition to the enthusiasm, even bravado, in this narrative, we are given a further sense of the aesthetic environment at Chottanikkara temple. The temple's large complex of shrines is carefully decorated and painted and spread over several acres of open grounds surrounded by hills. A variety of *pūjas* (worships) are carried out over the course of the day at the temple's shrines. Music is playing; incense is burning. In addition to the sensorial experience invoked by the environment of the temple, some of the mentally afflicted people at Chottanikkara report undergoing a spiritual change, a positive reorientation, or a movement to a state of health and well-being that is more auspicious than their pre-illness state. Recall Lakshmi, the woman introduced in Chapter 3 who was seeking Devi's assistance at Chottanikkara having previously tried allopathic treatment for her chronic fever, headache and fatigue. She described the healing process at Chottanikkara as an uplifting transformation:

> I have been coming to Chottanikkara for the last six years now. I came here because of the *chaitanyam* [power/consciousness] and blessing of the Devi [the goddess] at Chottanikkara. I started sitting for worship. From then until now, I haven't been to the hospital. I have no problem at all. I came here, and Devi changed everything for me. So I have been getting *aiśvaryam* [wealth/glory] and *abhivriddhi* [prosperity] continuously. Because of that blessing, I will be here forever.

While most patients talk of getting relief or change, Lakshmi speaks of receiving prosperity and blessing through healing. Although she claims to have overcome her problems, Lakshmi did not find a "cure," a simple ridding of her illness, and a return to health as a state of functionality. Rather, she feels she went through an auspicious transformation and developed a sense of well-being. "Health," or what one accomplishes in healing in this case, is not "remedial" (to borrow Alter's [1999] label for biomedical and anthropological assumptions about the nature of "health"). It is not a baseline state, absent of morbidity. It is something that can be constantly improved. Like the term *sukham* in Malayalam which means both "health" and "happiness" and is included in the everyday rhetorical question, "sukham ano?" ("Are you happy/healthy?" roughly akin to "How are you?"), it can be a state that is more vibrant and progressive than a simple absence of illness or presence of normal functionality.

Returning to the insights of Ajit, our most frequent interlocutor on ayurvedic therapy, we find an analogous claim to reach for "another level" of well-being through ayurveda. We recently heard of the difficulties Ajit experienced adapting to the requirements of the 45 day treatment at the Government Ayurveda Mental Hospital which necessitated that he stop smoking and change to a vegetarian diet. He said he grew to like the new regimen after a while, and later he commented on what he saw as contemporary views of health and the goals of allopathy and ayurveda. These comments, which introduced this study, merit revisiting:

> In the case of allopathic doctors, after asking two or three questions, they will know which medicine to prescribe. But ayurvedic doctors, they want to take the patient to another level. At that level, things are very different. Right now I am taking treatment for mental illness. For this illness, there is a painful method. It is giving "shocks." After going there and coming here [referring to allopathy and ayurveda], I feel this is better.

> [...]

> There might be some good aspects in allopathy when one looks at its research and other things, but if we want to get good *kulirmma* [coolness/satisfaction], if we want to reach a *nalla lakshyam* [good goal] . . . Right now, speaking about our life, what is it? If I have a fever, I must get better [literally: "must get changed"—*māranam*]. For what? To go for work the next day. Get a cold, get changed [*māranam*] in order to go to school the next day. This is the level at which we maintain our health. But if we have a supreme aim in life, ayurveda will help us attain it.

According to Ajit, ayurveda helps one to attain a "supreme aim," and as with Lakshmi, this involves a transformation rather than a simple removal of a problem. Ajit's views affirm Alter's (1999) claim, based on his reading of ayurvedic textual sources, that ayurvedic therapy aims at continual improvement of well-being, not just the resolution of problems of ill health.

In this excerpt, Ajit explains that a patient pursues *māranam* ("change," a form of the verb *māruka*), a goal that is more modest than the sense of eradication or return to normalcy in the allopathic concept of curing although it can also be seen as portending the larger, positive transformation Ajit says is possible. Some form of the verb *māruka* (to change) was used by many informants, including Kuttappan's wife above, to describe what was accomplished in healing. In a further attempt to explain her experience at Chottanikkara, Lakshmi added, "After some time, when we sat there, it felt like something was leaving from our body. It changed (*māri*) all our uneasiness. We were changing (*mārukayayirunnu*) in our selves." Here Lakshmi depicts her transformation during her first collective prayer experiences.

The uses of *māruka*/change can thus range from a description of incremental improvement to designating something like a "cure" (in labeling a more complete remission of illness) to indicating a more transcendent experience. In the excerpt above, Ajit adapts *māranam* to refer to a quick repair in order to be able to go to work or school the next day. This, he laments, is how we (an ambiguous "we" that could refer to people in Kerala but could be broader) conceive of our health today, and this kind of quick repair is a specialty of allopathy in the eyes of people in Kerala, a medical system that is especially attuned to contemporary work regimes and time constraints. In other words, Ajit laments that all "we" try to do nowadays is regain functionality.

Explanations and Implications

The abrasive effects of allopathic psychiatric treatments and the less uncomfortable, and occasionally pleasant, effects of ayurvedic treatments reported by current and former patients of these therapies may be due to ayurveda reinventing itself as a gentler alternative in the face of competition with allopathy. But this reinvention may in turn be enabled by epistemological and methodological orientations that inform these medical practices.

One could argue that allopathic medicine "thinks" in terms of disease *entities*, that behind every disease there is an identifiable cause which, if removed, would constitute a cure. Diseases have names such as cancer, malaria, depression or Attention Deficit Hyperactivity Disorder (ADHD) that confer essential, individual identities for afflictions. Some diseases, such as malaria or HIV, can be clearly identified by the presence of a distinct pathogen, but others such as ADHD or schizophrenia constitute a range on a continuum of behavior that is agreed upon by specialists. Allopathic practitioners are aware that some diseases do not have an identifiable cause—or they do not have one yet—and can only be healed by treating symptoms. However, where a cure is considered possible, a patient may be put through an unpleasant treatment in an effort to destroy a disease entity. This approach to "fighting" illness is reflected in the prolific use of war metaphors in biomedical discourse.[16] In fact, ECT has been described by psychiatrists as "a valued member of the treatment *armamentarium*" [my emphasis] for treating mental illness.[17] The metaphor of a war on a pathogen might be embraced, quite understandably, by people suffering HIV or malaria, but when the problem is psychological, psychiatric or spiritual—which allopathic psychiatry increasingly sees as being caused by biological agents—"attacking" the illness can be painful and problematic.

Ayurvedic medicine does not rely as heavily on the concept of disease entities. Disease categories exist in ayurveda, but often doctors address a specific constellation of symptoms in a particular patient and treat those particular symptoms and the humoral disturbances involved, frequently tailoring medications to particular patients' symptoms and bodily dispositions. Often, a patient is seen as someone who has a fever, dizziness and sleeping problems, rather than someone who has a particular disease that is indicated by these symptoms.[18] It is suggested here that such an orientation, toward treating the patient's discomforts through realigning and compensating bodily processes rather than destroying a pathogen, would lead one to consider how painful a process of treatment is. The process and the end result in such an orientation would likely be more palliative.

This patient-specific orientation may be declining in contemporary ayurvedic practice however. Formerly, I was told, the ayurvedic *vaidyan*—to use a classical name for an ayurvedic practitioner which is appropriate to this context—mixed a different medicine for each patient based on the patient's particular problems, and there are other ayurvedic physicians throughout Kerala who continue to apply this method in varying degrees. However, numerous ayurvedic pharmaceutical companies currently produce premixed, standardized medicines, and few *vaidyans* or suppliers can find the land or resources to keep a supply of the raw plant materials and other *materia medica* needed to create medicines at their practice. The use of standardized, pre-mixed medications may be leading to a propensity to treat disease entities rather than specific patient complaints.

It may seem a stretch to call on a literary analysis to help understand the workings of allopathy, but it is worth considering whether there is some epistemological affinity between the assumptions behind allopathic treatment and the end-oriented nature of western fiction observed by Frank Kermode (1967). Kermode claims that a sense of anticipating an ending, that originally stems from biblical accounts of the apocalypse, broadly underlies western fiction: "although for us the End has perhaps lost its naïve *imminence*, its shadow still lies on the crises of our fictions" (6). Kermode's examples from various periods, including modernist fiction demonstrate that authors narrate with a "sense of an ending" and an orientation to time that assumes an End. Allopathic treatment analogously appears to proceed while more firmly focused on an end goal of curing. It is perhaps this sense of an ending that leads "modern" people to rush and allopathic medicine to hurry—and thus overlook the quality of the process. We rush because time is short or limited as we approach the end. Benjamin Lee Whorf earlier made a similar point about the value of speed being linked to ideas about time that are inherent in European languages.[19] Of course, one could argue that a sense of an end is always present for all humans, not just those raised in an apocalyptic, Christian tradition, and it is not that the sense of an ending is necessarily lacking in ayurveda or religious healing (although Hindu cosmology does not anticipate an end of time). The difference may lie in the speed and the intensity with which ends are pursued. A determined focus on the goal of curing can obscure attention to the quality of the process of treatment while at the same time meeting the needs of people who themselves feel the pressure of time.

It is also possible that ayurvedic therapies are less abrasive to the body because ayurvedic medications are made from natural substances. Although these substances are refined and processed in factories, producers of ayurvedic medications do not isolate and create active chemical ingredients in laboratories as manufacturers of allopathic medicines do. A researcher at the state government-supported Tropical Botanical Garden and Research Institute explained to me that much is unknown about the effects on the body of chemical substances that naturally occur in plants, but it may be that potential side effects from naturally-occurring active chemical agents are mitigated by other, stabilizing "inactive" substances that coexist in a plant source. My conversations with this researcher, ayurvedic practitioners, and other specialists in plant pharmacognosy led me to develop the following rough distinction between allopathic and ayurvedic medications. Allopathic medications are made by producing isolated active chemical ingredients in laboratories. Drugs created in this manner provide greater dosages of chemical ingredients and produce more rapid effects while they also carry a greater risk of side effects. Medications made from plant materials have lower doses of active chemical ingredients and contain other, possibly stabilizing substances, which is why treatment in ayurveda takes longer and is perceived as less abrasive. I am not aware of any clinical studies that have tested the differences in rates of side effects between allopathic and ayurvedic medications, but the differences in the composition of these medications may help explain the distinction some people in Kerala make between fast-acting but dangerous allopathic drugs and slower, gentler ayurvedic medicines. This should not be taken to imply, however, that all ayurvedic medications are safe and properly prepared.[20]

Having called attention to concerns about the aesthetic experience of undergoing allopathic psychiatric procedures, it is important to remember that allopathy is the most frequently used form of psychiatric therapy in Kerala—although, as discussed earlier, it is difficult to quantify the availability of religious therapies for psychiatric problems. The popularity of allopathy relates partly to the fact that it is the most widely available psychiatric therapy system in Kerala, receiving the greatest investment from government and industry, but there is a particular virtue to this therapy that appealed to many patients and even competed with their concerns about the pleasantness of the process of therapy. Those who felt they could, or did, benefit from this therapy say that it can bring fast results, and many people we spoke to said they did not have the time to indulge in the more pleasant but more time-consuming therapy ayurveda offers. Although he yearned for loftier goals in treating illness, Ajit explained that allopathic treatment could fix a fever or other problems so that one could get back to work or school. Allopathy can help a person become functional again quickly so that he can return to his obligations. The idea of curing and health as remediation are thus appropriate to peoples' busy life-styles. Ganga, a Hindu woman who professes a faith in ayurvedic healing and whose in-laws are ayurvedic healers, was nevertheless receiving inpatient treat-ment at an allopathic psychiatric hospital for problems that included loss of consciousness, using abusive words toward her mother and problems eating. Ganga concurred with Ajit's view of allopathy which she says she uses for quick, temporary relief:

> Ganga: My husband's family is full of ayurvedic people, ayurvedic *vaidyans* [doctors]. My husband's father and uncle are *vaidyans*. So the whole family are vaidyans in ayurveda. So for quick [*pettennu*] relief only we came here. After this we will do ayurvedic treatment.

> Kavitha: You believe in that?

> Ganga: I very much believe in that. For immediate relief only we came here.

Ganga added that after she leaves the hospital she plans to use ayurvedic treatments at home with help from her husband and his family. Ganga and Ajit's observations represent tensions between the pleasantness and the speed of the healing process which raise compelling questions about pleasure, the nature of health and the speed of contemporary life.

Notes

1. For example, none of the articles in a volume called *Culture and Curing* (Morley and Wallis, eds. 1979) examines the concept of cure. It seems to be assumed that this is what the various healing systems discussed in the volume try to do in all contexts. Or, in an article called "Closure as Cure" (1986), Herzfeld explains that narrative closure in stories that are told by Greek healers help effect cure, in the sense of getting rid of a problem and returning to an original state of health. These works are highlighted here because the word "cure" appears prominently in their titles, but this term is regularly and casually used in many works of medical anthropology.
   As casual assumptions about curing are too frequent to review compre-hensively, I will mention just a few sources cited in other sections of this study that employ this concept uncritically. These examples should not be seen as espe-cially problematic uses of this concept but rather as typical examples of a regular

feature of medical anthropological writing (Bhattacharyya 1986: 47–49, Nichter and Nordstrom 1989: 384 and Roseman 1991: 9, 17, 129).

2. See, for example, Hahn and Gaines (1985), Payer (1988), B. Good and M. Good (1993), and specifically regarding the practice of psychiatry, Rhodes (1991) and Nunley (1996).

3. The literary examples from the Oxford dictionary for the first meaning of "cure" range from 1382 to 1623 while examples of the fifth definition range from 1526 to 1872, perhaps indicating a range of time when the sense of cure began to shift.

4. Hanks and Hoskin (1995), Redmond (1998).

5. Lipton and Cancro (1995: 971–985).

6. Callahan (1990); Morrison, Meier and Cassel (1996); Carney and Meier (2000).

7. Studies show rates of use of ECT in the United States at around 3% of psychiatric admissions between 1975 and 1986 and around 9% of patients with major depression in the early nineties (Rudorfer et al. 2003: 1867). Among my patient sample, the rate is around 5–10%. Nunley reports on his own and other researchers' findings that show the rate of ECT use in selected Indian hospitals ranges from 14% to 50% (1996: 168–169).

8. English-Malayalam dictionaries offer a variety of terms for the English "cure." However, these entries are usually long, Sanskritic neologisms, which translate into something like "to cause peace to come to an illness," and I did not observe these terms being used by informants (Mekkolla Parameswaran Pillai 1995, T. Ramalingam Pillai 1996).

9. Much to the point of this chapter, some Americans pay significant sums of money to receive this same *panchakarma* treatment for health maintenance and relaxation at ayurvedic-style health spas in Connecticut and New Mexico.

10. Most of the examples presented here come from fieldwork that was conducted in 1997. At that time, the GAMH was in a large, old, somewhat dilapidated house, an example of classic Kerala architecture that is often depicted in film and popular culture to represent a traditional image of hearth, home and Malayali identity. On returning to Kerala in 1999, I found that the GAMH had moved to a larger, modernist cement structure that resembled an allopathic hospital. I did not spend enough time at the new facility to thoroughly evaluate how it compared as an aesthetic environment for healing. There was more space inside the new hospital, yet treatments at this facility were administered indoors rather than outdoors. I couldn't help wondering to what degree modernizing this facility also involved imitating the architecture of biomedicine and perhaps losing a more aesthetically engaging environment.

11. Daniel (1984), Bhattacharyya (1986: 67), Nichter (1987) and Lamb (2000). Ram (1991) observed that in the Mukkuvar community (from a district of Tamil Nadu that borders Kerala) people are concerned about maintaining coolness and have many remedies for counteracting excessive heat. They are especially concerned about the accumulation of heat in the head and stress that one should apply copious amounts of cool water to the head when bathing (86).

12. Halliburton (2004).

13. This I did only partially so as not to be overly intrusive. For example, I observed (saw, heard and smelled) but did not participate in the dawn pujas and rituals at Chottanikkara temple. Like the mentally-afflicted devotees, my assistant Biju and I ate vegetarian food, which is said to be more calming and cooling, while

at Chottanikkara, but we did not eat with the devotees. I walked on the beach behind Vettucaud church after interviewing afflicted devotees, and I observed First Friday rituals (see Chapter 2). But I did not participate in prayers and rituals at the church.

14. It is problematic to compare a natural, but medicalized, bodily process (childbirth) to cases of psychopathology (though these could also be seen as "natural" developments), but these both involve situations for which a medical encounter is sought. Both myself and Van Hollen examined situations where medical intervention was sought, which Van Hollen points out is the case for most women giving birth in the region where she worked (56), and where a variety of options are available. This is neither an endorsement nor a critique of the medicalization of childbirth which Van Hollen depicts as both empowering and limiting.

15. For another example of healing systems responding to patient demands and preferences, see Scheid (2002) regarding Chinese and Western medicines in contemporary China.

16. Martin (1994).

17. Rudorfer et al. (2003: 1867).

18. The ayurvedic method of tailoring medications to specific patients has also been observed by Obeyesekere (1992).

19. In his classic comparison of Hopi and European languages, Whorf (1956[1939]) claims that because Europeans spacialize and quantify time, they think of time as something that can be wasted, and thus they value speed.

20. For a review of clinical studies of ayurvedic medications see (Khan and Balick 2001). A recent study reports heavy metal contaminants were found in 20% of ayurvedic medicines sampled, and illnesses have been reported from patients who used some of these medications (Saper et al. 2008). It is not clear whether this is part of an accepted practice among some ayurvedic practitioners or whether this is due to negligent preparation of these drugs.

6

༄

CONCLUSION: PLEASURE, HEALTH AND SPEED

At the end of the last chapter, I began to depict a simplified, but useful, dichotomy for understanding the changing meanings of the pleasantness of the process of treatment and what is accomplished in healing. People suffering mental afflictions who are able to choose between ayurvedic and allopathic treatments generally prefer the more pleasant process of treatment that ayurveda offers, yet many say they do not have the time, given their current work and lifestyle regimens, to indulge in the lengthier ayurvedic therapy. Thus people suffering mental afflictions in Kerala appear to be on the horns of a dilemma, negotiating between speed and pleasure in their healing choices, a dilemma that has profound implications for the quality of our health and our lives in the current (post)modern era.

Most people we interviewed described their problems, or those of afflicted family members, in terms of behaviors and mental and somatic symptoms, among the most common of which are sleeplessness, headache, outbursts of anger, refusing to eat and memory loss, and in many cases these symptoms were instigated by a vitiation of consciousness. In addition, several informants identified problems using English-language terms, including "tension" and "depression," that derive from professional and lay western psychological concepts and experiences.

Hanifa, the former Gulf migrant who was trying to cope with his "tension" at Beemapalli mosque, experienced problems including sleeplessness, running away from home and becoming easily distressed (*veprālam*—confused, worried), but in Hanifa and his wife's narratives, "tension" is the key term around which discussions of his problems revolve. In one of his first attempts to articulate his distress, Hanifa declared that "Something like a 'tension' has come." His wife added, "This 'tension' began when he was working in the Gulf. So he resigned from the job and came back." She also recalled that allopathic medicine caused him "memory problems and a lot of 'tension.'" Mary, the woman who wanted to become a nun and was being treated at the Government Ayurveda Mental Hospital after attempting suicide, also characterized her distress as involving "tension." In her first attempt to articulate her problems, Mary recalled "I got some mental 'tension'" (*"Enikku manassinu* tension *vannu"*).

Rajan, the Chottanikkara guest lodge employee who was formerly possessed at the temple, used an English-language idiom to describe the experience of possession. When a spirit enters the body or becomes active, one experiences fear, and "[t]hen what 'depression' we feel," he recalled. When asked how to tell when a possessing spirit has left, Rajan explained, "Problems like 'depression,' we are no longer getting anything like that."

The English term "stress" also arises in everyday conversation in Malayalam in Kerala, and handling "stress" has been the topic of psychological and psychiatric columns in popular magazines. Numerous conferences and workshops on stress management have been held in the state, including one organized by the University of Kerala Psychology Department in which I was asked to present a cultural anthropological account of stress. I chose to depict stress as an idiom that emerged in reaction to increased time pressure and accelerated time demands (Halliburton 1997).

The terms "tension," "depression" and "stress" evoke tactile, visceral images of physical pressure or torsion. "Stress" and "tension" also denote a sense of time pressure, a feature of contemporary life in Kerala that appears to relate to the popularity of allopathic therapy. Implicit in the concern for a pleasant process of therapy is an awareness of the unfolding, or the moment of passing (the "middest," in Kermode's terms [1967]), of time while the therapy is moving toward a goal of relief or transformation. But this way of viewing time erodes as people feel that they are constantly short of time. Sensing that life has sped up, they often turn to allopathic therapy when they are ill because, even if they do not like the process, the treatment does not require as great an investment of time as other options.

Reports of "stress" and time pressure are multiple and diffuse. Healers and friends in Kerala told me they lack sufficient time as they try to juggle the demands of work, school, family and social life. Keralites spend a significant portion of their early lives in school. Many pursue advanced degrees or special certificate programs and scramble for a better job. With the highest average number of years of schooling in India and a lack of jobs that are commensurate with their educational qualifications, people in Kerala feel they have to maximize their education, pursue private tutoring and earn the credentials they need to beat out other candidates for desirable jobs[1]. Computer training certificate programs are popular, and I often cringed at the pressure and expectations put on young people when I passed a banner advertisement in the middle- and working-class neighborhood where I lived enticing students to join a computer training program with "Want to emulate Bill Gates?"

When I visited Kerala in 1999, I was happy to learn that a friend and his wife had obtained coveted government sector jobs, which they had been seeking for years. However, like many Keralites who find their dream job, they had to pay a price in time and travel. My friend's job was in a city that, when the trains are running on time, was a two-hour commute from his home where he lives with his two sons. His wife, meanwhile, had begun working in northern Kerala, nine hours from their home, and she was able to visit only once every two weeks or so. When I saw this friend in the summer of 1999, he was waking up around 3:30 am to get his children ready for school and make it to his job on time. He would return home close to 7 pm, receive social and professional calls, help his sons with homework and, with luck, get to bed early enough to get four or five hours of sleep. Needless to say, he was always burnt out and yearning for more time. Upon learning of this couple's work situation, I became aware of others in similar circumstances. I was told that increasingly people commute four or more hours each way from Trivandrum to Cochin to work at a job that is commensurate with their skills or expectations. A small marketing niche was even forming around this new commuting pattern wherein food sellers jump onto the women's cars at the Cochin-Ernakulam train stations to sell vegetables and other groceries to female commuters who are still responsible for making dinner after their long journey home. When I last visited this couple in 2005, they had found jobs closer to home, but had taken on more responsibilities at work and appeared just as busy as before.

Osella and Osella's (2000a) ethnography of work and social aspirations among the Izhava caste (an upwardly-mobile, low caste, working class group) in a village in central Kerala provides similar observations about contemporary Kerala lifestyles and pressures. Izhavas align themselves with ideals of "progress" (this English term having been adopted into everyday Malayalam discourse) and put themselves under tremendous pressure to succeed in work and education in order to obtain consumer items and other symbolic capital that can help increase their social status. This keeps members of the Izhava caste quite busy, and time pressure is especially acute for working women who are expected to cook elaborate meals and carry out household duties after a long day of paid labor (38–46).

Not everyone is under the same time pressure, and this problem may vary by social class and profession. However, several patients and families I spoke to felt they could not afford to take the time to complete the 45-day treatment at the Government Ayurveda Mental Hospital or spend the weeks that are sometimes required to perform prayers and rituals at Chottanikkara temple. As we saw at the end of the last chapter, even Ganga, the daughter of a family of ayurvedic healers who holds ayurvedic therapy in high esteem, used allo-pathic treatment because she felt it would provide fast relief. These pressures, however, primarily affect the more functional patients who are not severely afflicted and have jobs or schooling to return to. Those individuals who are chronically ill and spend years in and out of hospitals, or reside at religious centers for extended periods, are unemployed or only occasionally employed and can be a great strain on families' time and resources.

These dilemmas do not seem limited to India. Farquhar (1994) touches on a similar issue in China, explaining that among Chinese urbanites who are otherwise attracted to Chinese medicine, "Young families no longer have an old grandmother handy to coordinate lots of elaborate cooking, and inten-sified work and study schedules leave little time to prepare and 'slowly sip' herbal decoctions" (476). Although people in these situations in China do not lament the loss of the kind of pleasant healing process I observed, those who use Chinese medicine do appreciate the thorough and aesthetically involved orientation to health and "looking at illness," to use Farquhar's translation of the Chinese term for what both doctor and patient do in the Chinese healing encounter (482). Furthermore, as mentioned in the discussion of Farquhar's work in Chapter 1, doctors of Chinese medicine do not work simply to remove symptoms, but rather, they aim for "a highly nuanced, positive, good health" (482). These are intriguing, but brief, incursions into these issues in the Chinese medical environment.[2] More research on the correlation between speed, health, aesthetics and work regimes in China and elsewhere would help us understand how widespread these dilemmas are and the degree to which they are linked to the introduction of biomedicine and changes in work regimens.

It is not only people suffering mental afflictions who have an opportunity to compare psychiatric healing systems that make the association between allopathic medicine and speed. Oxytocin drugs, which are in demand among expectant women in Tamil Nadu, speed up the process of childbirth while institutional constraints also lead doctors to use these medications to speed up the queue in hospitals (Van Hollen 2003). Van Hollen suggests that in crowded government hospitals in Chennai, where "rows upon rows of women lay right next to one another enduring the pain of early labor or recovering from delivery" (63), oxytocin drugs are employed "to keep women moving from the prenatal ward to the delivery ward to the postnatal ward and out in order to free up space for the steady influx of new women in labor" (64). Chapple (forthcoming) meanwhile demonstrates that in hospitals that are more devoted to "rescue"—intensive, heroic efforts to extend the life of people in critical condition—end-of-life palliative care can be affected by the clock time of the hospital and death can be treated as a goal and hastened. Doctors at rescue-intensive hospitals explain that a shorter time to death after patients are deemed beyond rescue, and a "do not resuscitate" (DHR) decision is made, reduces suffering for patients and families. Chapple questions whether dying should necessarily be seen as suffering and observes that at a community hospital that has fewer capacities to focus on and elaborate rescue, there is little concern that the post-DNR process of dying be quick—and she suggests the process of dying be used by family and friends to honor and say goodbye to the dying. Thus an emphasis on cure or rescue, and even the need of processing large numbers of patients, can speed up the process of treatment in allopathy.

Much has been made of E. P. Thompson's (1967) study of clock-time work discipline that he says emerged in Europe with industrial capitalism. The shift from task-oriented time (where workers work when tasks need to be completed) to clock time (where workers work for a certain number of hours measured by the clock) observed by Thompson has been associated with increased pressure on workers and a speeding up of industrial labor and productivity (Harvey 1990, Rubin 2007). Harvey (1990) examines what he and others see as an acceleration of life (work, tastes, fashions, methods of production and other aspects of everyday life) in the modern and postmodern periods. The modern period coincides with the advent of Fordist production in the workplace, and Harvey presents artists and intellectuals who lament the speeding up of life that accompanies these changes (260–283). The postmodern period that emerged in the late twentieth century is marked by strategies of flexible accumulation and organizational changes in production, such as "just in time" delivery and small-batch production, which "reduced turnover times in many sectors of production" and led to "an intensification (speed-up) in labour" (284–285). The speed of life, and especially the speed of change, has in turn accelerated in the postmodern era, which "accentuate[s] volatility and ephemerality of fashions, products, production techniques, labour processes, ideas and ideologies, values and established practices" (285).

The use of quick-fix treatments and an orientation to health as functionality (primarily in the workplace), rather than as the presence of well-being, certainly fits the current regimens of work and life described by Harvey. The time pressure people say they experience in Kerala, and the role of allopathic medicine as well as idioms of "tension" and "stress" in accommodating this, also support E. P. Thompson and David Harvey's insights about time and the pace of work and everyday life, but I have some hesitancy in celebrating an overly neat fit. While there have been cultural and economic transformations in India associated with industrialization and globalization, it would be inappropriate simply to apply Thompson and Harvey's analyses from Europe and North America to the context of India. Moreover, an association of time pressure with the advent of modern worklives in India would posit a past when people in India did not experience time pressure. Critiques of Thompson's depiction of clock time point to historical inaccuracies, claiming clock time long predates the work disciplines of the Industrial Revolution (Glennie and Thrift 2005), and demonstrate that other methods of measuring time created clock-time style work discipline in the medieval period (Birth 2009). In other words, a past that was lacking in time pressure seems somewhat idealized, and while the worklife and workplace temporalities research has little to say about changes in time disciplines in India,[3] I doubt that premodern, precolonial work and lifestyle regimens were lacking in time pressures. One does not need a clock or a "modern" job to feel such pressure. This can develop through multiple, overlapping tasks and constantly emerging work, family and life obligations (the latter of which are more acute in "traditional" extended families [Rudolph, Rudolph and Kanota 2000]). The situation may actually be that people have long felt time pressure from work and other obligations, but when ayurveda is the primary treatment option, it is simply accepted that one must take weeks off to treat a significant illness. Once allopathy becomes available as a faster option for treatment (probably after the pharmaceutical turn in the mid-twentieth century), people are able to choose this option and return to their obligations sooner. This may then lead to more normative pressures and expectations to return to work quickly, which then may be reinforced by modern and developmentalist ideologies of productivity and speed.

Whether contemporary lifestyles involve greater time pressure, which makes allopathy more appealing, or the availability of allopathy creates greater expectations of speed and productivity, the use of allopathy to quickly return to obligations raises the issue of how "health" is perceived, engaged and lived out. Recalling Ajit's lament—"Get a cold, get changed in order to go to school the next day. This is the level at which we maintain our health"—completing therapy to the extent that one can return to one's obligations and productivity, shapes an orientation to health as functionality. Concerns about this approach to health, rather than engaging health as positive transformation, recall the insights of early social critics of medicine including Rudolf Virchow (1958) and Ivan Illich (1976), who linked modern standards of health and illness to life and work conditions under capitalism, and the not-yet-realized World Health Organization (1978) definition of health as not simply the absence of disease but also the presence of a state of well-being. People suffering mental problems in Kerala reveal a continuum of dispensations including the intriguing possibility of going beyond a cure and achieving an auspicious state of transformation that is more enhanced than their pre-illness state. The latter orientation ultimately differs from the WHO ideal of health as the presence of well-being, which itself may be on the wane.[4] While the WHO position is more positive than the absence-of-pathology view of health, it retains the sense of health as a state of stasis, as achieving and then maintaining a state of well-being. For some patients in Kerala and in Alter's (1999) interpretation of ayurvedic texts, health is a process of constant improvement or constant growth. With such a definition, however, "health" begins to lose its adequacy as a description of the aspirations involved, and perhaps we are considering broader goals of life which can be achieved, in part, through therapy. Ajit alludes to a goal that transcends our usual sense of health, healing and what is accomplished in medical realms when he claims that ayurveda can help one attain a "supreme aim in life." Similarly, Lakshmi asserts she has "been getting *aiśvaryam* [wealth/glory] and *abhivriddhi* [prosperity] continuously" through her relationship with the goddess at Chottanikkara.

These are of course heady ideals for health and the quality of life. Perhaps Lakshmi and Ajit will have trouble maintaining these aspirations. Perhaps they will relapse and struggle again to find some "change," as many do in coping with mental adversity. They and others experiencing mental distress at least expose us to orientations to "health" that many of us who live in a more medically homogeneous society remain unaware of since we are attuned to our common-sense assumptions, which are shaped by biomedical discourses and practices. Having had the chance to compare different psychiatric treatments, people in Kerala know that there are multiple options and multiple dilemmas: some therapies are more pleasant than others, some are faster than others and some claim they can help one aim for another level of health.

Marcus and Fischer (1999) assert that one of the primary purposes of anthropology should be cultural critique. One should be able to use the insights from comparing cultural practices to critically re-evaluate one's own cultural assumptions (the culture to be critiqued in their examples is the "West," or roughly European and North American ideologies and practices). People who live in a medically pluralistic environment are essentially natural anthropologists of medical practice due to their experience comparing and critiquing approaches to healing. This development of an evaluative, critical perspective is inevitable as patients and their families navigate and compare medical options bearing in mind their concerns about suffering, healing and aesthetic experience. In an effort to improve approaches to health and healing, biomedical practitioners, and really anyone who is concerned about health, should consider the critical insights offered by those in Kerala who have observed and compared different systems of healing and use these to improve their therapeutic techniques.

Although some in privileged cosmopolitan enclaves in less medically diverse settings, such as the United States, do pursue health as constant improvement through often expensive spa-like health centers and "alternative" healing and health maintenance sessions and retreats, this orientation to health is considered a privilege and is not widely accessible. The problem for people in more medically homogeneous societies lies in the lack of broadly available options and the lack of diverse models for configuring new approaches to health. Any change in this situation would necessitate grand changes in people's worklives and the nature of our fast and stressful (post)modern society. And in the United States, where even a right to basic biomedical health care has not yet been realized, it is hard to imagine a broad-based promotion of "pleasurable" alternatives and transcendent ideals of health. The practices of people and of the state in Kerala, where wealth and material resources are far less plentiful, though, demonstrate that "pleasant" healing options need not be confined to those who can afford spas and high-end alternative medical treatments. I noted earlier the irony that the *panchakarma* treatment (involving enemas, nasally administered medicines and other procedures described in Chapter 2) which is provided free to patients at Kerala's Government Ayurveda Mental Hospital is also available at significant cost at ayurvedic health centers in New England and New Mexico.

Such ayurvedic care need not be made available and affordable everywhere, and it would be wrong to suggest that biomedicine should downplay the importance of its many vital invasive procedures and life-saving drugs, even if these do have unpleasant side effects. But, especially in the realm of mental health, biomedical practitioners might use these insights into the pleasantness of the healing process to enhance the aesthetic experience of biomedical psychiatric treatment. Something akin to this has been achieved in the world of obstetrics as observed in the most recent edition of Emily Martin's now classic critique of biomedical child-birthing practices, *The Woman in the Body* (2001). Although undergoing childbirth may never be a pleasant process, some hospitals give women multiple options for labor and delivery and create an aesthetically engaging environment. A 2008 article in *The Atlantic Monthly* reports links between better aesthetic design in hospital interiors and improved patient health and—recalling patients in Kerala who left allopathic therapy to pursue more pleasant forms of treatment—observes that women have changed obstetricians to deliver in hospitals with aesthetically-pleasing, hotel-like birthing centers (Postrel 2008). Similar reforms deserve serious consideration in the world of psychiatric care where dramatic procedures such as electroconvulsive therapy continue to be experienced as unpleasant, even punitive, measures and the aesthetic drabness of biomedical institutional environments does not add to the morale of the mentally afflicted and depressed.

Patients in Kerala also alert us to the possibility of thinking of health as constant improvement or "healing" as an opportunity to progress through an illness to a state that is more enhanced than one's pre-illness state. Meanwhile, the Malayalam practice of referring to what is accomplished in therapy as experiences of "change" attends to the subtle, incremental character of "healing" a mental illness and may in fact be necessary for seeing the process of healing as a balancing act between the goals of therapy and the quality of the process of undergoing treatment. These insights hopefully will influence mental health practitioners to further attend to the visceral quality of the treatment process while pursuing the goals of therapy. They should also compel us to ask whether our contemporary work and lifestyle regimens have been leading us to give up pleasantness for the sake of speed and whether we forgo other orientations to health because our late capitalist world resigns us to see health as being merely functional. These problems require remedies that go beyond suggestions for the aesthetic design of healing centers and the avoidance of abrasive healing techniques. For now, they will hopefully lead to further critical consideration of how to balance productivity, health and well-being.

Notes

1. On the level of education see National Family Health Survey-India (1995:53) and on underemployment see Mathew (1997).
2. The politics of aesthetics and sensory experience in China are explored in more detail in Farquhar (2002), although the focus is primarily on food and sexuality. Nevertheless, as Farquhar observes, these realms link to the aesthetic engagements of Chinese medicine.
3. Other than recent global outsourcing work (Poster 2007), which has little relation to the lives of most people I met in Kerala.
4. A review of more recent reports by the WHO (2007a, 2007b) did not reveal explicit affirmations of this orientation to health, which may be symptomatic of an increasingly hegemonic view of health as a return to functionality.

Appendix A

SEMI-STRUCTURED INTERVIEW QUESTIONS

(Where and when interview took place and name of assistant is noted.)
Speaker (s): [e.g., patient, patient's mother, spouse etc.]

Biographical/Demographic

1) Where are you from? [Where is your "sthalam"?]
2) What is your occupation? For how long?
3) What is your age?
4) What is highest level of education you have attained?

Illness/Affliction

5) What is the problem for which you are seeking treatment?
6) What bothers you most about this problem? What are your current symptoms?
7) Is this the first treatment you have sought for this problem? For example, have you sought help from a temple, an astrologer, ayurveda, allopathy or anywhere else?

If answer to question 7 is "no," go to question 8. If "yes" go to question 11.

8) (If previous treatment was different therapy) why did you change therapies? or are you still using the previous therapy in addition to the current one?

9) Did you experience the same symptoms during the previous therapy? Have you experienced any new symptoms or feelings since beginning the current therapy?

10) Did you/do you agree with how previous and current therapists saw your problem?

Social Implications

11) Has this problem caused you any social inconvenience or financial hardship?

12) Has your difficulty caused any family tensions?

Nature and Prognosis of Problem

13) What do you think has been the cause of your problem? Have you always felt that this is the cause? If not, how have your views changed?

14) What do you think needs to be done to end your affliction/illness?

15) What specific plan do you have to end your affliction/illness? How long will this take? What is the next step you will take?

REFERENCES

Alter, Joseph
1999 Heaps of Health, Metaphysical Fitness: Ayurveda and the Ontology of Good Health in Medical Anthropology. *Current Anthropology* 40: 43–66.

American Library Association-Library of Congress
1997 *ALA-LC Romanization Tables: Transliteration Schemes for Non-Roman Scripts.* Washington, D.C.: Library of Congress.

Arnold, David
2000 *Science, Technology and Medicine in Colonial India.* Cambridge, UK: Cambridge University Press.

Augé, Marc
1999[1994] *An Anthropology for Contemporaneous Worlds.* Stanford, CA: Stanford University Press.

Baer, Hans, Merrill Singer and Ida Susser
2004 *Medical Anthropology and the World System: Second Edition.* Westport, CT: Praeger.

Battaglia, Debbora
1995 Problematizing the Self: A Thematic Introduction. In *Rhetorics of Self-Making.* Debbora Battaglia, ed. Pp. 1–15. Berkeley: University of California Press.

Bhattacharyya, Deborah
1986 *Pāgalāmi: Ethnopsychiatric Knowledge in Bengal.* Syracuse, NY: Maxwell School of Citizenship and Public Affairs, Syracuse University.

Birth, Kevin
2009 Illiteracies of the Imagination, Necromantic Devices and How Clocks Make Us Stupid. Paper presented at Guggenheim Museum exhibition on time. New York, NY, January 7.

Black's Medical Dictionary
1992 *Black's Medical Dictionary—37th Ed.* Lanham, MD: Barnes & Noble Books.

Boddy, Janice
1989 *Wombs and Alien Spirits: Women, Men, and the Zar Cult in Northern Sudan.* Madison: University of Wisconsin Press.

Bordo, Susan
1993 *Unbearable Weight: Feminism, Western Culture and the Body.* Berkeley: University of California Press.

Bourguignon, Erika
1991 *Possession.* Prospect Heights, IL: Waveland Press.

Brodwin, Paul
1996 *Medicine and Morality in Haiti: The Contest for Healing Power.* Cambridge, UK: Cambridge University Press.

Brooks, Douglas Renfrew
1992 *Auspicious Wisdom: The Texts and Traditions of Śrīvidyā Śākta Tantrism in South India.* Albany, NY: SUNY Press.

Bruner, Edward
1986 Experience and Its Expressions. In *The Anthropology of Experience.* V. Turner and E. Bruner, eds. Pp. 3–32. Urbana, IL: University of Illinois Press.

Callahan, Daniel
1990 *What Kind of Life? The Limits of Medical Progress.* New York: Simon and Schuster.

Caraka
1998 *Caraka Samhitā.* R.K. Sharma and Bhagwan Dash, eds. Varanasi: Chowkhamba Sanskrit Series Office.

Carney, M. T. and Diane E. Meier
2000 Palliative Care and End-of-Life Issues. *Anesthesiology Clinics of North America* 18(1): 183–209.

Carstairs, G. M. and R. L. Kapur
1976 *The Great Universe of Kota: Stress, Change and Mental Disorder in an Indian Village.* Berkeley: University of California Press.

Cassel, Eric
1982 The Nature of Suffering and the Goals of Medicine. *New England Journal of Medicine* 306(11): 639–645.

Chapple, Helen
Forthcoming *Death With as Little Dying as Possible.* Walnut Creek, CA: Left Coast Press.

Climent, C. E., B. S. M. Diop, T. W. Harding, H. H. A. Ibrahim, L. Ladrido-Ignacio and N. N. Wig
1980 Mental Health in Primary Care. *WHO Chronicle* 34: 231–236.

Cohen, Lawrence
1998 *No Aging in India: Alzheimer's, the Bad Family, and Other Modern Things.* Berkeley: University of California Press.

Crandon-Malamud, Libbet
1993 *From the Fat of Our Souls: Social Change, Political Process, and Medical Pluralism in Bolivia.* Berkeley: University of California Press.

Csordas, Thomas
1990 Embodiment As A Paradigm for Anthropology. *Ethos* 18: 5–47.
1993 Somatic Modes of Attention. *Cultural Anthropology* 8(2): 135–156.
1994 Introduction: The Body as Representation and Being-in-the-World. In *Embodiment and Experience: The Existential Ground of Culture and Self.* Thomas Csordas, ed. Pp. 1–26. Cambridge, UK: Cambridge University Press.
1999 The Body's Career in Anthropology. In *Anthropological Theory Today.* Henrietta Moore, ed. Pp. 172–205. Cambridge, UK: Polity Press.

Dale, Stephen F.
1990 Trade, Conversion and the Growth of the Islamic Community of Kerala, South India. *Studia Islamica* 71: 155–175.

Daniel, E. Valentine
1984 *Fluid Signs: Being a Person the Tamil Way.* Berkeley: University of California Press.

Dash, Vaidya Bhagwan and Acarya Manfred Junius
1983 *A Handbook of Ayurveda.* New Delhi: Concept Publishing Company.

Desai, Manali
2005 Indirect British Rule, State Formation, and Welfarism in Kerala, India, 1860–1957. *Social Science History* 29(3): 457–488.

Desjarlais, Robert
1992 *Body and Emotion: The Aesthetics of Illness and Healing in the Nepal Himalayas.* Philadelphia: University of Pennsylvania Press.
1997 *Shelter Blues: Sanity and Selfhood Among the Homeless.* Philadelphia: University of Pennsylvania Press.

Devi, R. Niranjana
2006 *Medicine in South India.* Chennai: Eswar Press.

Devisch, René
1993 *Weaving the Threads of Life: The Khita Gyn-Eco-Logical Healing Cult Among the Yaka.* Chicago: University of Chicago Press.

Doyle, Derek, Geoffrey Hanks and Neil MacDonald
1998 Introduction. In *Oxford Textbook of Palliative Medicine—Second Edition.* Derek Doyle, Geoffrey Hanks, and Neil MacDonald, eds. Pp. 3–10. New York: Oxford University Press.

Dumont, Louis
1970[1966] *Homo Hierarchichus: The Caste System and Its Implications.* Chicago: University of Chicago Press.
1986[1983] *Essays on Individualism: Modern Ideology in Anthropological Perspective.* Chicago: University of Chicago Press.

Eck, Diana
1998 *Darśan: Seeing the Divine Image in India—3rd Edition.* New York: Columbia University Press.

Estroff, Sue E.
1981 *Making It Crazy: An Ethnography of Psychiatric Clients in an American Community.* Berkeley: University of California Press.

Ewing, Katherine
1991 Can Psychoanalytic Theories Explain the Pakistani Woman? Intrapsychic Autonomy and Interpersonal Engagement in the Extended Family. *Ethos* 19(2): 131–161.
1997 *Arguing Sainthood: Modernity, Psychoanalysis and Islam.* Durham, NC: Duke University Press.

Fabian, Johannes
1983 *Time and the Other: How Anthropology Makes Its Object.* New York: Columbia University Press.

Farmer, Paul
1992 The Birth of the *Klinik*: A Cultural History of Haitian Professional Psychiatry. In *Ethnopsychiatry: The Cultural Construction of Professional and Folk Psychiatries.* Atwood Gaines, ed. Pp. 251–272. Albany: SUNY Press.

Farquhar, Judith
1994 Eating Chinese Medicine. *Cultural Anthropology* 9(4): 471–497.
2002 *Appetites: Food and Sex in Post-Socialist China.* Durham, NC: Duke University Press.

Fishburn, Katherine
1997 *The Problem of Embodiment in Early African American Narrative.* Westport, CT: Greenwood Press.

Forero-Peña, Alcira
2004 To Stand on Their Own: Women's Higher Education in Kerala, India. Ph.D. dissertation. Department of Anthropology. The Graduate Center—City University of New York.

Foundation for the Revitalization of Local Health Traditions
2006 Encyclopedia of Indian Medicinal Plants. Available at: http://www.frlht.org.in/meta Accessed: October 17, 2008.

Franke, Richard W. and Barbara H. Chasin
1994 *Kerala: Radical Reform as Development in an Indian State—Second Edition.* Oakland, CA: Institute for Food and Development Policy.
2000 Is the Kerala Model Sustainable? Lessons from the Past, Prospects for the Future. In *Kerala: The Development Experience.* Govindan Parayil, ed. Pp. 16–39. London: Zed Books.

Fuller, C.J.
1992 *The Camphor Flame: Popular Hinduism and Society in India.* Princeton, NJ: Princeton University Press.

Geertz, Clifford
1986 Making Experience, Authoring Selves. In *The Anthropology of Experience*. V.
      Turner and E. Bruner, eds. Pp. 373–380. Urbana, IL: University of Illinois
      Press.

Ghosh, Amitav
1992 *In an Antique Land: History in the Guise of a Traveler's Tale*. New York: Vintage.

Gilbert, Pamela
1997 *Disease, Desire and the Body in Victorian Women's Popular Novels*. Cambridge, UK:
      Cambridge University Press.

Glennie, Paul and Nigel Thrift
2005 Revolutions in the Times: Clocks and the Temporal Structures of Everyday Life.
      In *Geography and Revolution*, D. Livingstone and C.Withers, eds., Pp. 160–98.
      Chicago: University of Chicago Press.

Good, Byron
1994 *Medicine, Rationality and Experience: An Anthropological Perspective*. Cambridge,
      UK: Cambridge University Press.

Good, Byron J. and Mary-Jo DelVecchio Good
1993 "Learning Medicine:" The Constructing of Medical Knowledge at Harvard
      Medical School. In *Knowledge, Power and Practice: The Anthropology of Medicine
      and Everyday Life*. Shirley Lindenbaum and Margaret Lock, eds. Pp. 81–107.
      Berkeley: University of California Press.

Gough, Kathleen
1959 The Nayars and the Definition of Marriage. *Journal of the Royal Anthropological
      Institute* 89: 23–34.
1968 Literacy in Kerala. In *Literacy in Traditional Societies*. Jack Goody, ed. Pp. 132–
      160. Cambridge, UK: Cambridge University Press.

Govinda Pillai, P.
1999 Lecture on social history of Kerala. University of Wisconsin Kerala Summer
      Program. Trivandrum, Kerala. June 26.

Gulati, L.
1983 Male Migration to the Middle-East and the Impact on the Family: Some
      Evidence from Kerala. *Economic and Political Weekly* 18(52–53): 2217–2226.

Gupta, Satya Pal
1977 *Psychopathology in Indian Medicine (Āyurveda)*. Aligarh, India: Ajaya Publishers.

Habib, S. Irfan and Dhruv Raina
2005 Reinventing Traditional Medicine: Method, Institutional Change, and the
      Manufacture of Drugs and Medication in Late Colonial India. In *Asian
      Medicine and Globalization*. Joseph Alter, ed. Pp. 67–77. Philadelphia: University
      of Pennsylvania Press.

Hahn, Robert and Atwood Gaines
1985 *Physicians of Western Medicine: Anthropological Approaches to Theory and Practice*.
      Dordrecht: D. Reidel Publishing.

Halliburton, Murphy
1997 Stress As an Idiom of Social Change. Paper presented at Conference on Stress and Stress Management, sponsored by Department of Psychology, University of Kerala. Thiruvananthapuram (Trivandrum), Kerala, India.
1998 Suicide: A Paradox of Development in Kerala. *Economic and Political Weekly* 33(36–37): 2341–2345.
2004 Finding a Fit: Psychiatric Pluralism in South India and Its Implications for WHO Studies of Mental Disorder. *Transcultural Psychiatry* 41(1): 80–98.
2005 "Just Some Spirits:" The Erosion of Spirit Possession and the Rise of 'Tension' in South India." *Medical Anthropology* 24(2): 111–144.
In press Drug Resistance, Patent Resistance: Indian Pharmaceuticals and the Impact of a New Patent Regime. *Global Public Health.*

Hanks, G. W. and P. J. Hoskin
1995 Pain and Symptom Control in Advanced Cancer. In *Oxford Textbook of Oncology.* M. Peckham, H. Pinedo, and U. Veronesi, eds. Pp. 2417–2430. Oxford: Oxford University Press.

Harding T. W., M. V. de Arango, J. Baltazar, C. E. Climent, H. H. Ibrahim, L. Ladrido-Ignacio, R. S. Murthy and N. N. Wig
1980 Mental Disorders in Primary Health Care: A Study of Their Frequency and Diagnosis in Four Developing Countries. *Psychological Medicine* 10: 231–241.

Harvey, David
1990 *The Condition of Postmodernity: An Enquiry into the Origins of Cultural Change.* Cambridge, MA: Blackwell.

Herzfeld, Michael
1986 Closure as Cure: Tropes in the Exploration of Bodily and Social Disorder. *Current Anthropology* 27(2): 107–120.

The Hindu (articles by unnamed staff reporters)
1997 1,306 to Get Gulf War Compensation. April 10.

Illich, Ivan
1976 *Medical Nemesis: The Expropriation of Health.* New York: Pantheon Books.

Jackson, Michael
1996 Introduction. In *Things As They Are: New Directions in Phenomenological Anthropology.* Michael Jackson, ed. Pp. 1–50. Bloomington, IN: Indiana University Press.

Janzen, John
1978 *The Quest for Therapy: Medical Pluralism in Lower Zaire.* Berkeley: University of California Press.

Jecker, Nancy S. and Donnie J. Self
1991 Separating Care and Cure: An Analysis of Historical and Contemporary Images of Nursing and Medicine. *Journal of Medicine and Philosophy* 16: 285–306.

Kakar, Sudhir
1982 *Shamans, Mystics and Doctors: A Psychological Inquiry into India and Its Healing Traditions.* Chicago: University of Chicago Press.

Kapferer, Bruce
1983 *A Celebration of Demons: Exorcism and the Aesthetics of Healing in Sri Lanka.* Bloomington, IN: Indiana University Press.
1997 *The Feast of the Sorcerer: Practices of Consciousness and Power.* Chicago: University of Chicago Press.

Kaplan, Harold and Benjamin Sadock
1995 *Comprehensive Textbook of Psychiatry—Sixth Edition.* Baltimore: Williams & Wilkins.

Kavitha N.S.
1996 Stressors and Stress Coping Among Wives of Gulf Expatriates. M.A. Thesis. Department of Psychology. University of Kerala, Thriuvananthapuram.

Kehoe, Alice and Dody Giletti
1981 Women's Preponderance in Possession Cults: The Calcium-Deficiency Hypothesis Extended. *American Anthropologist* 83: 549–561.

Kermode, Frank
1967 *The Sense of an Ending: Studies in the Theory of Fiction.* New York: Oxford University Press.

Khan, Sarah and Michael J. Balick
2001 Therapeutic Plants of Ayurveda: A Review of Selected Clinical and Other Studies for 166 Species. *Journal of Alternative and Complementary Medicine* 7(5): 405–515.

Kirschner, Suzanne
1996 *The Religious and Romantic Origins of Psychoanalysis: Individuation and Integration in Post-Freudian Theory.* Cambridge, UK: Cambridge University Press.

Kleinman, Arthur
1980 *Patients and Healers in the Context of Culture.* Berkeley: University of California Press.
1986 *Social Origins of Distress and Disease: Depression, Neurasthenia and Pain in Modern China.* New Haven, CT: Yale University Press.
1988a *Rethinking Psychiatry: From Cultural Category to Personal Experience.* New York: Free Press.
1988b *The Illness Narratives: Suffering, Healing and the Human Condition.* New York: Basic Books.

Kleinman, Arthur, Veena Das and Margaret Lock
1997 *Social Suffering.* Berkeley: University of California Press.

Kleinman, Arthur and Joan Kleinman
1995 Suffering and Its Professional Transformation: Toward an Ethnography of Interpersonal Experience. In *Writing at the Margins: Discourse Between Anthropology and Medicine.* Pp. 95–119. Berkeley: University of California Press.

Kleinman, Arthur and Lilias Sung
1979 Why Do Indigenous Practitioners Successfully Heal? *Social Science and Medicine* 13B: 7–26.

Kline, Nathan S.
1954 Use of Rauwolfia Serpentia Benth in Neuropsychiatric Conditions. *Annals of the New York Academy of Sciences* 59: 107–132.

Kothari, Manu L. and Lopa A. Mehta
1988 Violence in Modern Medicine. In *Science, Hegemony and Violence: A Requiem for Modernity*. Ashis Nandy, ed. Pp. 167–210. Delhi: Oxford University Press.

Kusserow, Adrie Suzanne
1999 Crossing the Great Divide: Anthropological Theories of the Western Self. *Journal of Anthropological Research* 55: 541–562.

Laderman, Carol and Marina Roseman
1996 Introduction. In *The Performance of Healing*. Carol Laderman and Marina Roseman, eds. Pp. 1–16. New York: Routledge.

Lakoff, George and Mark Johnson
1980 *Metaphors We Live By*. Chicago: University of Chicago Press.
1999 *Philosophy in the Flesh: The Embodied Mind and Its Challenge to Western Thought*. New York: Basic Books.

Lamb, Sarah
2000 *White Saris and Sweet Mangoes: Aging, Gender and Body in North India*. Berkeley: University of California Press.

Langford, Jean
1998 Ayurvedic Psychotherapy: Transposed Signs, Parodied Selves. *Political and Legal Anthropology Review* 21(1): 84–98.
2002 *Fluent Bodies: Ayurvedic Remedies for Postcolonial Imbalance*. Durham, NC: Duke University Press.

Leslie, Charles
1976 The Ambiguities of Medical Revivalism in Modern India. In *Asian Medical Systems: A Comparative Study*. Charles Leslie, ed. Pp. 356–367. Berkeley: University of California Press.
1992 Interpretations of Illness: Syncretism in Modern Ayurveda. In *Paths to Asian Medical Knowledge*. Charles Leslie and Alan Young, eds. Pp. 177–208. Berkeley: University of California Press.

Lewis, Ioan M.
1983 Spirit Possession and Biological Reductionism: A Rejoinder to Kehoe and Giletti. *American Anthropologist* 85: 412–413.
1989 *Ecstatic Religion: A Study of Spirit Possession and Shamanism—Second Edition*. London: Routledge.

Lipton, Alan and Robert Cancro
1995 Schizophrenia: Clinical Features. In *Comprehensive Textbook of Psychiatry—6th Edition*. Harold Kaplan and Benjamin Sadock, eds. Pp. 968–987. Baltimore: Williams & Wilkins.

Lock, Margaret
1993 Cultivating the Body: Anthropology and Epistemologies of Bodily Practice and Knowledge. *Annual Review of Anthropology* 22: 133–155.

Madhavanpillai, C.
1976 *Malayalam English Nighandu*. Kottayam: National Book Stall.

Mani, V.S.
1998 Major Mental Health Issues in Kerala. Paper. Kerala Mental Health Authority. Thiruvananthapuram.

Mankekar, Purnima
1999 *Screening Culture, Viewing Politics: An Ethnography of Television, Womanhood and Nation in Postcolonial India*. Durham, NC: Duke University Press.

Marcus, George and Michael Fischer
1999 *Anthropology as Cultural Critique: An Experimental Moment in the Human Sciences—Second Edition*. Chicago: University of Chicago Press.

Marriott, McKim
1976 Hindu Transactions: Diversity Without Dualism. In *Transaction and Meaning: Directions in the Anthropology of Exchange and Symbolic Behavior*. Bruce Kapferer, ed. Pp. 109–142. Philadelphia: Institute for the Study of Human Issues.
1989 Constructing an Indian Ethnosociology. *Contributions to Indian Sociology* 23(1): 1–39.

Marsella, Anthony and Geoffrey White, eds.
1982 *Cultural Conceptions of Mental Health and Therapy*. Dordrecht: D. Reidel Publishing Company.

Martin, Emily
1994 *Flexible Bodies: Tracking Immunity in American Culture From the Days of Polio to the Age of AIDS*. Boston: Beacon Press.
2001 *The Woman in the Body: A Cultural Analysis of Reproduction*. Boston: Beacon Press.

Mathew, E.T.
1997 *Employment and Unemployment in Kerala: Some Neglected Aspects*. New Delhi: Sage.

Maya, C.
2006 Poor Delivery of Mental Health Services in State. *The Hindu*. July 3. http://www.hindu.com/2006/07/03/stories/2006070309820500.htm. Accessed April 9, 2007.

Mencher, Joan
1965 The Nayars of South Malabar. In *Comparative Family Systems*. M.N. Nimkoff, ed. Pp. 163–191. New York: Houghton Mifflin Co.

Merleau-Ponty, Maurice
1962 *Phenomenology of Perception*. New York: Humanities Press.

Meulenbeld, G. Jan.
1999 *A History of Indian Medical Literature—Volume 1A*. Groningen, Netherlands: Egbert Forsten.

Mines, Mattison
1988 Conceptualizing the Person: Hierarchical Society and Individual Autonomy in India. *American Anthropologist* 90: 568–579.

Morley, Peter and Roy Wallis, eds.
1979 *Culture and Curing: Anthropological Perspectives on Traditional Medical Beliefs and Practices*. Pittsburgh: University of Pittsburgh Press.

Morrison, R. Sean, Diane E. Meier and Christine K. Cassel
1996 When Too Much Is Too Little. *New England Journal of Medicine* 335(23): 1755–1759.

Mosby's Medical, Nursing & Allied Health Dictionary
2002 *Mosby's Medical, Nursing & Allied Health Dictionary—6th Ed.* St. Louis: Mosby (Elsevier Science).

Mullings, Leith
1984 *Therapy, Ideology, and Social Change: Mental Healing in Urban Ghana*. Berkeley: University of California Press.

Nabokov, Isabelle
2000 *Religion Against the Self: An Ethnography of Tamil Rituals*. New York: Oxford University Press.

Nadkarni, Vital
1997 Brahmi Rediscovered. *Times of India*. Feb. 16.

Nair, Sunitha B.
2001 Social History of Western Medical Practice in Travancore: An Enquiry into the Administrative Process. In *Disease and Medicine in India: A Historical Overview*. Deepak Kumar, ed. Pp. 215–232. New Delhi: Tulika Books.

Narayanan, M. G. S. et al.
1976 *Kerala Through the Ages*. Thiruvananthapuram: Government of Kerala Department of Public Relations.

National Crime Records Bureau (Government of India)
1994 *Accidental Deaths and Suicides in India*. New Delhi: Ministry of Home Affairs.

National Family Health Survey
1995 *National Family Health Survey—Kerala 1992–3*. Bombay: International Institute for Population Studies. Thiruvananthapuram: Population Research Centre, University of Kerala.

Nichter, Mark
1981 Idioms of Distress: Alternatives in the Expression of Psychosocial Distress: A Case from South India. *Culture, Medicine and Psychiatry* 5: 379–408.
1987 Cultural Dimensions of Hot, Cold and Sema in Sinhalese Health Culture. *Social Science and Medicine* 25(4): 377–387.

Nichter, Mark and Carolyn Nordstrom
1989 A Question of Medicine Answering: Health Commodification and the Social Relations of Healing in Sri Lanka. *Culture, Medicine and Psychiatry* 13: 367–390.

Nirmala, K.A.
1997 Levels of Mortality and Social Development in Kerala and Andhra Pradesh: A Comparative Perspective. Paper presented at Dr. T.N. Krishnan Memorial

Seminar on Development Experience of South Indian States in a Comparative Setting. Thiruvananthapuram: Centre for Development Studies. 7–9 September.

Nunley, Michael
1996 Why Psychiatrists in India Prescribe So Many Drugs. *Culture, Medicine and Psychiatry* 20: 165–197.
1998 The Involvement of Families in Indian Psychiatry. *Culture, Medicine and Psychiatry* 22: 317–353.

Obeyesekere, Gananath
1982 Science and Psychological Medicine in the Ayurvedic Tradition. In *Cultural Conceptions of Mental Health and Therapy*. A. Marsella and G. White, eds. Pp. 235–248. Dordrecht: D. Reidel Publishing Co.
1985 Depression, Buddhism and the Work of Culture in Sri Lanka. In *Culture and Depression: Studies in the Anthropology and Cross-cultural Psychiatry of Affect and Disorder*. Arthur Kleinman and Byron Good, eds. Pp. 134–152. Berkeley: University of California Press.
1992 Science, Experimentation and Clinical Practice in Ayurveda. In *Paths to Asian Medical Knowledge*. Charles Leslie and Allan Young, eds. Pp. 160–176. Berkeley: University of California Press.

Olfson, Mark, Steven Marcus, Harold A. Sackeim, James Thompson and Harold Alan Pincus
1998 Use of ECT for the Inpatient Treatment of Recurrent Major Depression. *American Journal of Psychiary* 155: 22–29.

Ong, Aihwa
1987 *Spirits of Resistance and Capitalist Discipline: Factory Women in Malaysia*. Albany, NY: SUNY Press.

Osella, Filippo and Caroline Osella
2000a *Social Mobility in Kerala: Modernity and Identity in Conflict*. London: Pluto Press.
2000b Migration, Money and Masculinity in Kerala. *Journal of the Royal Anthropological Institute* (N.S.) 6: 117–133.

Oxford English Dictionary
1933[1972 Supplement] *Oxford English Dictionary*. Vol. II, C. (Plus *A Supplement to the Oxford English Dictionary*. Vol. I, A-G) Oxford University Press.

Pandolfi, Mariella
1993 Le *Self*, le corps, la <<crise de la présence.>> *Anthropologie et Sociétés* 17(1–2): 57–78.

Panikar, P.G.K. and C.R. Soman
1984 *Health Status of Kerala: Paradox of Economic Backwardness and Health Development*. Thiruvananthapuram: Centre for Development Studies.

Parayil, Govindan, ed.
2000 *Kerala: The Development Experience*. London: Zed Books.

Parry, Jonathan
1989 The End of the Body. In *Fragments for a History of the Human Body—Part Two*. Michel Feher, Ramona Naddaff and Nadia Tazi, eds. Pp. 491–517. New York: ZONE.

Payer, Lynn
1988 *Medicine and Culture: Varieties of Treatment in the United States, England, West Germany and France*. New York: H. Holt.

Pfleiderer, Beatrix
1983 Words and Plants: A Concept of Ayurvedic Psychotherapy. *Sociologus: Zeitschrift fur Empirische Ethnosoziologie und Ethnopsychologie [A Journal for Empirical Ethno-sociology and Ethno-psychology]* (Berlin) 33(1): 25–41.
1988 The Semiotics of Ritual Healing in a North Indian Muslim Shrine. *Social Science and Medicine* 27(5): 417–424.

Piccinelli, Marco and Gregory Simon
1997 Gender and Cross-Cultural Differences in Somatic Symptoms Associated with Emotional Distress. An International Study in Primary Care. *Psychological Medicine* 27: 433–444.

Pillai, Mekkolla Parameswaran
1995 *Assissi English-Malayalam Dictionary*. Changanacherry: Assissi Printing and Publishing House.

Pillai, T. Ramalingam
1996 *English-English-Malayalam Dictionary*. Kottayam: D. C. Books.

Pollock, Donald
1996 Personhood and Illness among the Kulina. *Medical Anthropology Quarterly* 10(3): 319–341.

Poster, Winifred
2007 Saying "Good Morning" in the Middle of the Night: The Reversal of Work Time in Globalized ICT Service Work. In *Workplace Temporalities* (special monograph edition of *Research in the Sociology of Work* 17), Beth A. Rubin, ed. Pp. 55–112. Amsterdam: Elsevier.

Postrel, Virginia
2008 The Art of Healing. *The Atlantic Monthly* 301 (3): 119–122.

Prabodhachandran Nayar, V. R.
1994 Malayalam. In *Encyclopedia of Language and Linguistics*. Ronald Asher, ed. Pp. 2350–2351. Oxford: Pergamon Press.

Quashie, Kevin Everod
2004 *Black Women, Identity and Cultural Theory: (Un)Becoming the Subject*. New Brunswick, NJ: Rutgers University Press.

Radhakrishnan, Sarvepalli and Charles Moore, eds.
1957 *A Sourcebook in Indian Philosophy*. Princeton, NJ: Princeton University Press.

Ram, Kalpana
1991 *Mukkuvar Women: Gender, Hegemony and Capitalist Transformation in a South Indian Fishing Community.* London: Zed.

Ramachandran, V. K.
2000 Kerala's Development Achievements and Their Replicability. In *Kerala: The Development Experience.* Govindan Parayil, ed. Pp. 88–115. London: Zed Books.

Redmond, Kathy
1998 Treatment Choices in Advanced Cancer: Issues and Perspectives. *European Journal of Cancer Care* 7(1): 31–39.

Rhodes, Lorna A.
1991 *Emptying Beds: The Work of an Emergency Psychiatric Unit.* Berkeley: University of California Press.

Roland, Alan
1988 *In Search of the Self in India and Japan: Toward a Cross-Cultural Psychology.* Princeton, NJ: Princeton University Press.

Romanucci-Ross, Lola
1969 The Hierarchy of Resort in Curative Practices: The Admiralty Islands, Melanesia. *Journal of Health and Social Behavior* 10: 201–209.

Roseman, Marina
1991 *Healing Sounds From the Malaysian Rainforest: Temiar Music and Medicine.* Berkeley: University of California Press.

Rubin, Beth A.
2007 Time-Work Discipline in the 21st Century. In *Workplace Temporalities*, (special monograph edition of *Research in the Sociology of Work* 17). Beth A. Rubin, ed. Pp. 1–26. Amsterdam: Elsevier.

Rudolph, Susanne, Lloyd Rudolph and Mohan Singh Kanota
2000 *Reversing the Gaze: Amar Singh's Diary—A Colonial Subject's Narrative of Colonial India.* New Delhi: Oxford University Press.

Rudorfer, Matthew, Michael Henry and Harold Sackeim
2003 Electroconvulsive Therapy. In *Psychiatry—Second Edition.* Allan Tasman, Jerald Kay, and Jeffrey Lieberman, eds. Pp. 1865–1901. Chichester, UK: John Wiley & Sons, Ltd.

Saith, Ashwani
1992 Absorbing External Shocks: The Gulf Crisis, International Migration Linkages and the Indian Economy, 1990 (with Special Reference to the Impact on Kerala). *Development and Change* 23: 101–146.

Śankaracharya
1973 [orig. 8th century] *Upadeśa Sāhasrī.* Translated by Swami Jagadananda. Madras: Sri Ramakrishna Math.

Saper, Robert B., Russell Phillips, Anusha Sehgal, Nadia Khouri, Roger Davis, Janet Paquin, Venkatesh Thuppil and Stefanos Kales
2008 Lead, Mercury, and Arsenic in US- and Indian-Manufactured Ayurvedic Medicines Sold via the Internet. *JAMA* 300(8): 915–923.

Scheid, Volker
2002 *Chinese Medicine in Contemporary China: Plurality and Synthesis.* Durham, NC: Duke University Press.

Scheper-Hughes, Nancy
1992 *Death Without Weeping: The Violence of Everyday Life in Brazil.* Berkeley: University of California Press.

Scheper-Hughes, Nancy and Margaret Lock
1987 The Mindful Body: A Prolegomenon to Future Work in Medical Anthropology. *Medical Anthropology Quarterly* 1: 6–41.

Selby, Martha Ann
2005 Sanskrit Gynecologies in Postmodernity: The Commoditization of Indian Medicine in Alternative Medical and New-Age Discourses on Women's Health. In *Asian Medicine and Globalization.* Joseph Alter, ed. Pp. 120–131. Philadelphia: University of Pennsylvania Press.

Sen, G. and K.C. Bose
1931 Rauwolfia Serpentina: A New Indian Drug for Insanity and High Blood Pressure. *Indian Medical World* 11: 194–201.

Sharp, Lesley
1994 Exorcists, Psychiatrists, and the Problem of Possession in Northwest Madagascar. *Social Science and Medicine* 38(4): 525–542.

Shweder, Richard
1991 *Thinking Through Cultures: Expeditions in Cultural Psychology.* Cambridge, MA: Harvard University Press.

Shukla, G. D.
1989 Electro-Convulsive Therapy: A Review. *Indian Journal of Psychiatry* 31(2): 97–115.

Sivarajan, V. V. and Indira Balachandran
1994 *Ayurvedic Drugs and Their Plant Sources.* New Delhi: Oxford & IBH Publishing.

Skultans, Vieda
1991 Women and Affliction in Maharashtra: A Hydraulic Model of Health and Illness. *Culture, Medicine and Psychiatry* 15(3): 321–359.

Sreedhara Menon, A.
1990 *Kerala History and Its Makers—Second Edition.* Madras: S. Viswanathan Publishers Pvt., Ltd.

Srivastava, Sanjay
2005 *Ghummakkads,* a Woman's Place, and the LTC-*walas*: Towards a Critical History of "Home," "Belonging" and "Attachment." *Contributions to Indian Sociology* 39(3): 375–405.

Strathern, Andrew
1996 *Body Thoughts*. Ann Arbor, MI: University of Michigan Press.

Thomas Isaac, T.M.
1997 Economic Consequences of Gulf Migration. In *Kerala's Demographic Transition: Determinants and Consequences*. K. C. Zachariah and S. Irudaya Rajan, eds. Pp. 269–309. New Delhi: Sage.
2000 Making of the Kerala Model of Development: The Role of Public Policy and Social Movements. Paper presented to the Department of Anthropology and Howard Samuels Center, CUNY Graduate Center, New York, NY. February 9.

Thomas Isaac, T.M., Richard Franke and Pyaralal Raghavan
1998 *Democracy at Work in an Indian Industrial Cooperative: The Story of Kerala Dinesh Beedi*. Ithaca, NY: Cornell University Press.

Thompson, E. P.
1967 Time, Work-Discipline, and Industrial Capitalism. *Past and Present* 38: 56–97.

Udayan, P.S., K.V. Tushar and Satheesh George
2007 A New Variety of *Humboldtia* (Fabaceae: Caesalpinioideae) from the Western Ghats of India. *Journal of the Botanical Research Institute of Texas* 1(1): 121–127.

Vaidyanathan, K. R.
1988 *Temples and Legends of Kerala*. Bombay: Bharatiya Vidya Bhavan.

Vaidyanathan, T. G.
1989 Authority and Identity in India. *Daedalus* 118: 147–169.

Van Hollen, Cecilia
2003 Invoking *Vali*: Painful Technologies of Modern Birth in South India. *Medical Anthropology Quarterly* 17(1): 49–77.

Varier, Vaidyaratnam P. S.
1996 *Chikitsa Samgraham*. Kottakkal, India: Arya Vaidya Sala.

Virchow, Rudolf
1958 *Disease, Life and Man: Selected Essays*. Lelland Rather, trans. Stanford, CA: Stanford University Press.

Waldman, Amy
2003 Gulf Bounty Is Drying Up in Southern India. *New York Times*. Feb. 24, p.A3.

Weiner, James
1997 Ethnology. In *Encyclopedia of Phenomenology*. Lester Embree, ed. Pp. 198–202. Dordrecht: Kluwer Academic Publishers.

Weiss, Mitchell
1986 History of Psychiatry in India: Toward a Culturally and Historiographically Informed Study of Indigenous Traditions. *Samiksa* 40(2): 31–45.

Weiss, Mitchell, S. D. Sharma, R. K. Gaur, J. S. Sharma, A. Desai and D. R. Doongaji
1986 Traditional Concepts of Mental Disorder Among Indian Psychiatric Patients: Preliminary Report of Work in Progress. *Social Science and Medicine* 23(4): 379–386.

Weiss, Mitchell, Amit Desai, Sushrut Jadhav, Lalit Gupta, S. M. Channabasavanna, D. R. Doongaji and Prakash B. Behere
1988   Humoral Concepts of Mental Illness in India. *Social Science and Medicine* 27(5): 471–477.

Whorf, Benjamin Lee
1956[1939] The Relation of Habitual Thought and Behavior to Language. In *Language, Thought and Reality: Selected Writings of Benjamin Lee Whorf*. Pp. 134–159. Cambridge, MA: MIT Press.

Wilce, James
1998   *Eloquence in Trouble: The Poetics and Politics of Complaint in Rural Bangladesh.* New York: Oxford University Press.
2004   Madness, Fear and Control in Bangladesh: Clashing Bodies of Power/ Knowledge. *Medical Anthropology Quarterly* 18(3): 357–375.

Wikan, Unni
1991   Toward an Experience-Near Anthropology. *Cultural Anthropology* 6: 285–305.

World Health Organization (WHO)
1978   *Primary Health Care.* Geneva: World Health Organization.
2007a *The World Health Report 2007—A Safer Future: Global Public Health Security in the 21ˢᵗ Century.* Geneva: World Health Organization. Available at http://www. who.int/whr/2007/en/. Accessed July 23, 2008.
2007b *Working for Health: An Introduction to the World Health Organization.* Geneva: World Health Organization. Available at http://www.who.int/about/. Accessed July 23, 2008.

Young, Allan
1995   *The Harmony of Illusions: Inventing Post-Traumatic Stress Disorder.* Princeton, NJ: Princeton University Press.

Young, James C.
1981   *Medical Choice in a Mexican Village.* New Brunswick, NJ: Rutgers University Press.

Zimmermann, Francis
1987   *The Jungle and the Aroma of Meats: An Ecological Theme in Hindu Medicine.* Berkeley: University of California Press.
1992   Gentle Purge: The Flower Power of Āyurveda. In *Paths to Asian Medical Knowledge.* Charles Leslie and Allan Young, eds. Pp. 209–224. Berkeley: University of California Press.
1995   The Scholar, the Wise Man, and Universals: Three Aspects of Ayurvedic Medicine. In *Knowledge and the Scholarly Medical Traditions.* Don Bates, ed. Pp. 297–319. Cambridge, UK: Cambridge University Press.

INDEX

Advaita Vedānta philosophy, 143
agriculture, 24
allopathic hospitals, 60, 62–63
allopathic medicines, 59, 64–66;
    composition of, 190; experience
    taking, 117–18, 131–32;
    fluoxetine, 65; haloperidol, 64–65,
    135n5; Hexidol, 99, 135n5; side
    effects of, 118, 159, 178
allopathic treatment, 58–66; aesthetic
    experience of, 12, 176–77, 202;
    availability of, 62, 190; compared
    with ayurvedic treatment, 11–12,
    55, 66, 161, 167–68, 177–78,
    180; counseling in, 57; goals of,
    13–14, 189; inpatient care in,
    66; outpatient care in, 63–66;
    palliative care in, 166–67;
    reactions to, 167–68, 175–77;
    speed of, 14, 116, 189,
    190–91, 195
allopathy, 11, 34, 36n1, 42, 58–66;
    compared with ayurveda,
    43–44; concept of cure in,
    160; concept of time in, 162,
    189; disease entities in, 188;
    hegemony of, 155, 181; history
    in India of, 59–60; in colonial

and postcolonial period, 181;
    popular media discourses of, 15;
    promotion of, 60
Alter, Joseph, 13, 20, 46–47, 164, 186,
    187, 201
alternative medicine, 43
Amma-Narayana (divinity), 67. *See also*
    Chottanikkara temple
Arnold, David, 59
Arya Vaidya Sala, 48, 51, 60
Ashram, Divy Shanti, 84
astrology, 85
ati (hit, spank, slap or beat), 107–09
ātman (intangible, true self, soul), 18,
    30, 142–43, 147, 162. *See also*
    experience, modes of
ayurveda, 11, 34, 41–42;
    commodification of, 48;
    compared with allopathy,
    43–44; concept of time in, 162;
    disease entities in, 188–89;
    features of, 45–48; in colonial
    and postcolonial period, 181;
    in other parts of the world, 48;
    medical texts in, 43–44; origins
    of, 60; philosophy of, 44, 49;
    popular media discourses of,
    156; promotion of, 60; purism in,

ABOUT THE AUTHOR

Murphy Halliburton is tenured assistant professor of anthropology at Queens College and the Graduate Center, City University of New York. His specialities are medical anthropology, anthropology of science and South Asian culture and history.